CHOOSING A NURSING HOME

SETH B. GOLDSMITH

PRENTICE
HALL
PRESS

NEW YORK·LONDON·TORONTO·SYDNEY·TOKYO·SINGAPORE

PRENTICE HALL PRESS
15 Columbus Circle
New York, NY 10023

Library of Congress Cataloging-in-Publication Data

Goldsmith, Seth B.
    Choosing a nursing home / by Seth B. Goldsmith. — 1st Prentice
Hall Press ed.
      p.   cm.
    Includes bibliographical references.
    ISBN 0-13-298779-1
    1. Nursing homes.   2. Aged — Institutional care — Decision making.
I. Title.
RA997.G65   1990
362.1′6 — dc20   89-48844
                                           CIP

Designed by Robert Bull Design

Manufactured in the United States of America

10 9 8 7 6 5 4 3 2 1

First Edition

Dedicated to
Sandra
Jonas and Benjamin

ACKNOWLEDGMENTS

This book would not have been possible without the assistance of numerous people. To all of these individuals, particularly the ones who are inadvertently not mentioned, I am grateful.

First, I want to thank Jean Drewsen, my agent, and PJ Dempsey, my initial editor at Prentice Hall Press, who both were supportive of this project from the outset and helpful in the initial shaping of the book. Following PJ's departure from Prentice Hall, I was fortunate to have my book come under the guidance of editors Paul Aron and David Dunton, both of whom provided useful ideas, excellent technical support, and the right amount of encouragement.

Special thanks also go to Howard Braverman, who was always available to answer my queries about any aspect of nursing homes or provide me with the latest regulation or other document about long-term-care facilities.

Next I would like to acknowledge the many long-term-care professionals who so generously provided me with their personal and professional hospitality by opening their organizations (and sometimes their houses), organizing site visits in their communities, and frequently being available for what must have seemed like endless telephone consultations: Moe Brown, Mel Weisman, Stan Schiffman, Al Mendlovitz, Sol Goldner, George Geisin, Sharon Sizemore, Herbert Shore; and Denny Magid, Miriam Parker, Bryan Mesh, Irv Kronenberg, Brad Morton, Sheldon Blumenthal, Kent Kirkwood, Bob Burmeister, Dick Lamben, Marvin Goldberg, Bill Ihle, Bill Mathies, Harvey Shankman, Jim Reich, Kathleen Reinke,

Bruce Arneil, Alvan Small, Joshua Gortler, Drew Gackenheimer, Mary Jo Pompeo, Marvin Neuman, Bill Compton, Lynn Craft, Pat McMurray, Mark Forman, Marie-Louise Ansak, Edna Green, Richard Huddy, Gail MacLean, Maury May, Michael Weinfeld, Franklin Williams, Don Gilmore, Bob Johnson, Robert Freestate, Jeanette Isenberg, Cheryl Eubanks, Ziva Itzenberg, Claire Kearns, Judy Bennett, Pat Scruffle, Susan Bryer, Irving Hoff, Fredlee Shore, Herman Sabrsula, Ron Tardiff, Carol Farrington, Larry Knowles, Stephen Russo, Lois Gackenheimer, Mark Ponder, Steve Raichilson, Harvey Young, Wesley Sperr, Jonathan Hyde, Vicki Luman, Merlin Southwick, Henry Rosenberg, Frank Sansom, Steve Roisin, Helen Norris, and Anne Arakaki-Lock.

I would also like to thank the scores of nursing-home residents and their families who shared with me their personal stories about nursing-home life.

Thanks go to my mother, Ida Goldsmith, and my father-in-law, Irving Brooks, who assisted my efforts by regularly sending me articles they clipped from their Florida and Texas newspapers.

I received other valuable assistance from my dean at the University of Massachusetts School of Public Health, Dr. Stephen H. Gehlbach, who encouraged my work on this project, accompanied me on several site visits, and provided helpful criticism of an early draft of this book.

My two sons, Jonas and Benjamin, also deserve a special acknowledgment for their interest in this project, consistent good humor, and forbearance while I was on the road. Finally, I want to thank my wife, Sandra, who provided me with the crucial emotional and essential logistical support that I needed in order to write this book.

CONTENTS

PREFACE

The starting point for my research for this book may have been a visit in the early 1960s to a Brooklyn, New York, nursing home, where my eighty-year-old maternal grandfather spent the last months of his life in a hot, crowded ward that stank with the smell of urine. I was about twenty at the time and did not quite understand why he had moved out of the small room in which he had lived for so many years at an aunt's house—a room with a stack of Yiddish newspapers, his collection of pipes, and the familiar pungent odor of Prince Albert tobacco. Almost thirty years later, I still do not quite understand what happened.

Although the trauma of that visit probably kept me away from the interiors of nursing homes for many years, I became active in the nursing-home industry via other avenues. My academic posts—first at Tulane University in New Orleans and later at Columbia University in New York and the University of Massachusettts in Amherst—provided me with myriad opportunities to teach health-care management to both novice and fully licensed nursing-home administrators. The teaching generated some small research projects that eventually found their way into the professional literature.

In the mid-1970s, I had the good fortune to be appointed to the New York State Board of Examiners for Nursing Home Administrators—the official body that has the responsibility for setting and enforcing the standards for administrators. The work of the board usually was mundane, although on occasions (such as license revocation hearings) it rose to the level of high drama. In thinking back over my experiences on the board, I realize that the issues with which I had to wrestle in those days provided me with a perspective on the nursing-home industry that was important and different from the one I had developed from the vantage point of the ivory tower.

In 1987, I had another occasion to study nursing homes at close range. This unique opportunity came in the form of a fellowship from the Association of University Programs in Health Administration, funded by the Princeton, New Jersey–based Robert Wood Johnson Foundation. The fellowship allowed me to spend several months working full time as an in-house senior consultant to a 200-bed not-for-profit intermediate and skilled-nursing facility.

From the moment I walked through the front door of that nursing home, I knew that it was significantly different from the facility to which my grandfather had been relegated. Residents were out of bed and dressed; many were obviously perky; therapy rooms were bustling with activity; an activities program offered something more than bingo; a physician was in attendance on a full-time basis; there was obviously a caring attitude on the part of the staff; and the place did not smell of urine. During the course of my fellowship, I met with residents and their families, interviewed staff, studied regulations, observed the operations of the facility, interviewed board members and administrators, and watched the ebb and flow of life in a nursing home, with its inevitable highs and lows. By the time I completed the fellowship, I had become convinced that, despite the myriad problems of nursing-home financing and regulation, it was still possible to deliver high-quality, sensitive care to nursing-home residents.

A short time later, I decided to become a nursing-home activist on the community level. For example, I was elected to the board of a not-for-profit nursing home, where I presently serve as vice-president, chairman of the Marketing Committee, and a member of the Planning Committee. At the University of Massachusetts School of Public Health, where I serve as Professor of Health Policy and Management, I introduced materials on nursing homes into all of my courses and developed a new graduate course on issues in long-term-care policy and management. At my law firm, Bowditch and Dewey in Worcester, Massachusetts, I made the affairs of nursing homes the prime focus of my legal practice. Finally, I decided to pose the following question to myself: What does it take to make an excellent nursing home?

To answer this question, I thoroughly studied the professional and popular literature, but, most important, I visited all manner of nursing homes—from coast to coast and in between—searching for examples of excellent nursing homes. By the time I finished this project, I had covered 40,000 miles and visited a broad range of homes in twenty-three states. These facilities included homes that were privately owned, others that were under the aegis of governmental agencies, and a number that were managed by a variety of private, not-for-profit fraternal and religious groups. Hundreds of people, including elderly nursing-home residents, nurses, physicians, administrators, owners, trustees, and government officials, were kind enough to share with me their experiences and analyses of nursing-home life.

All of these varied exposures to both poor-quality and excellent nursing homes inevitably resulted in this book, which is neither an exposé of nursing homes nor an apologia for the nursing-home industry. Rather, it focuses on assisting potential nursing-home residents and their families to sort through the complex issues facing them in evaluating and selecting a nursing home. It is a book that applauds America's excellent nursing homes, encourages consumers to demand more of the homes, and, above all, tries to persuade the nursing-home industry to do better by our country's elderly.

INTRODUCTION: THE WORLD OF NURSING HOMES

Nobody thinks that going into a nursing home is going to happen to them. . . . Nobody prepares themselves for this. They think they are going to live forever the way they are living.

—Mr. S. F., eighty-year-old
nursing-home resident, Louisville, Kentucky

Each year, 1.3 million elderly people are admitted to the 20,000 nursing homes in the United States. Typical of these new residents is Mrs. L., who, as a seventy-eight-year-old widow, moved from her nephew's large and comfortable suburban home into a Massachusetts nursing home. In thinking about the decision to move, she recalled that "It was my decision more or less but it was a compromise; my nephew had three children growing up and because of my trouble walking and occasional dizziness, they had to get someone to stay with me if their friends invited them over but didn't invite me. I decided that this move would be best for me." Mrs. L.'s story is similar to those of the more than 500,000 people who each year move into nursing homes from their own residences or those of family and friends. Almost every one of these people will spend the remainder of their lives in the nursing home. Typically, these new residents are white, widows, more than seventy-five years of age, and require assistance in bathing, dressing, toileting, eating, and getting in and out of bed and chairs. Mrs. L. was among the fortunate ones who had both the time and the energy to participate with other family members in the evaluation and selection of her new home.

Every year, another 500,000 people are transferred directly

from hospitals to nursing homes. When such a transfer is required, the family is likely to be under considerable pressure to select a nursing home within forty-eight hours. For some of these patients, the nursing home is merely a way station on their road home—less expensive than a hospital for recuperating and receiving rehabilitative services. For most of these patients, the stay may last a few weeks or months, but they eventually leave the institution and return to a more traditional mode of living. However, a significant number of these 500,000 transferees will become permanent nursing-home residents who never return to their previous homes and rarely, despite plans to the contrary, transfer to another nursing home.

The selection of a nursing home is confusing, complex, time-consuming, and ridden with anxiety. Additionally, the burden of the decision and the research necessary to make a good choice fall squarely on the shoulders of the family and the potential resident. Physicians—the professionals we usually rely on to be our surrogate decision-makers on health matters—frequently know little about the range of nursing-home possibilities in a region, and rarely have they invested the time to comparison-shop several facilities.

Pressure for making a quick decision may also be generated by the hospital, which is caught in a conflict of interest between its objective of transferring a patient out of the institution's unreimbursed $750-a-day bed and the needs of the patient and his or her family. The fiscal reality is that the faster the hospital effects the transfer, the more money it makes or saves on the patient. Along with this, the hospital staff orchestrating this transfer is likely to be more interested in finding a vacant nursing-home bed as soon as possible than in finding the best placement for the long haul. In some instances, the hospital staff will have only limited information about local nursing homes, and, perhaps because of the enormous pressure of their jobs, they may have neither visited the homes they are recommending nor performed any evaluation or follow-up studies of their placements.

On the other hand, some hospital social workers, discharge planners, or local physicians may be of enormous help in identifying alternatives and making suggestions. But since the final decision is a personal one with the long-run implications equal to those of moving into a new abode in a new town, it should not be finessed to a stranger. Finally, because of the elderly person's condition, the family members inevitably are forced into the difficult position of investigating, evaluating, and selecting the nursing home. In order to negotiate this nursing-home labyrinth and make an informed as well as a good choice, the initial step is to become an educated consumer. Necessarily, this education must begin in chapter 1 with a basic understanding of the language of nursing homes and some of the key issues of ownership and staffing. In chapter 2, I shall take several different perspectives to examine the issue of the need for nursing-home services. Chapter 3 considers the alternatives to nursing homes, such as New York State's "Nursing Home Without Walls" program, the "On Lok" system in San Francisco, home care, and others. Chapters 4 and 5 look at different aspects of paying for nursing-home care. These chapters examine the important public financing programs of Medicare and Medicaid, the private long-term-care insurance question, and finally the hidden costs of nursing-home care. In chapter 6, I provide an overview of the quality of care in nursing homes and follow this in chapter 7 with information on how to measure quality. Chapters 8 and 9 delineate the tasks and steps a family or potential resident should follow in selecting a nursing home. These chapters are filled with guides for action. Chapter 10 provides a summary and a final analysis of what constitutes an excellent nursing home. Throughout this volume, the reader will encounter actual people, facilities, and programs from which much can be learned.

ONE

NURSING-HOME BASICS

TERMINOLOGY BASICS:
Medicare, Medicaid, SNFs, ICFs, and RCFs.

Many of the rules and regulations having the greatest impact on what happens in individual nursing homes are requirements generated by the Medicare and Medicaid programs. Medicare is the federally financed program, primarily for the over–sixty-five population. It was, and to a great extent still is, a hospital insurance program. In various attempts to cut the high costs associated with in-hospital care, Medicare has allowed payment for hospital substitutes, such as home-health-care services and nursing-home care. Originally, many of these out-of-hospital benefits required a prior hospital stay. For the short life of the Medicare Catastrophic Coverage Act of 1988, which was implemented on January 1, 1989, and repealed in November of 1989, many elderly people became eligible to have Medicare pay their nursing-home bill. However, before Medicare would pay the bill, it was required that the resident receive an intense level of skilled or rehabilitative care under a doctor's supervision and the nursing-home bed be Medicare-certified (frequently only several beds in a nursing home or only part of a home may be certified for Medicare). Unfortunately this has resulted in a government-sanctioned and disruptive game of musical beds with nursing homes shifting residents around the home into and out of Medicare beds based on the availability of funds and beds. With the repeal of the Catastrophic Act it is anticipated that we will go back to the prior system by which Medicare rarely paid for long-term nursing-home care.

The Medicaid program that pays for nursing-home care is a state and federal partnership designed to care for a variety of groups, particularly the medically needy. While the federal government does have a number of restrictions for these programs, each state has considerable authority to tailor its program, so there are enormous regional variations in nursing-home reimbursements. Texas, for example, pays in the neighborhood of $35 per day to care for Medicaid recipients, while Connecticut pays closer to $150 per day for Medicaid-eligible residents. Perhaps of greater significance is the rigorousness with which the states monitor the care delivered to Medicaid recipients. This subject is covered in the chapters on quality of care.

A nursing home—or, in some cases, units in a nursing home—generally is classified as one of three types of facilities: skilled-nursing facilities (SNFs); intermediate-care facilities (ICFs); or residential-care facilities (RCFs). Basically, these three classifications are a reflection of the intensity of services required by the residents and offered by the facilities.

The distinctions between skilled-nursing and intermediate-care nursing homes and services are often hard to understand because there is a broad spectrum of state and federal definitions and requirements. Further confusing matters is one section of the Omnibus Budget Reconciliation Act of 1987, which was signed by President Ronald Reagan on December 22, 1987, containing a provision that for Medicaid payment purposes eliminates the distinctions between skilled-nursing and intermediate-care facilities and introduces a new term into the health-care lexicon: "nursing facility" (NF). The meaning of this is simple: Regardless of what Medicaid pays for, the same standards must be met.

Medicare, however, is very specific with regard to its requirements for skilled-nursing care. It requires that the skilled-nursing services for which it pays (1) be ordered by a physician; (2) be so inherently complex that the services must be provided by and under the supervision of technical or professional health personnel, such as nurses, physical therapists, or speech pathologists; (3) be required on a daily basis; and (4) be furnished for a condition that arose as a result of a recent hospitalization.

It is often difficult to understand the meaning of various Medicare definitions and regulations. In a respectable attempt to clarify its own ambiguous regulations, Medicare provides several examples of what type of clinical situation qualifies for Medicare-financed skilled-nursing or rehabilitation services. One example:

> An aged patient with a history of diabetes mellitus and angina pectoris who is recovering from an open reduction of the fracture of the neck of the femur requires, among other services, careful skin care, appropriate oral medications, a diabetic diet, an exercise program to preserve muscle tone and body condition, and observation to detect signs of deterioration in his or her condition or complications resulting from restricted, but increasing, mobility.

Medicare acknowledges that any one of the services required by this hypothetical person could be provided by a caregiver who had been given proper instruction. However, despite this acknowledgment, it concludes that for the aged diabetic person with chest pains to receive the care that ensures recovery, it will be necessary to have a skilled professional, presumably a nurse, plan and manage the patient's care. According to Medicare, this planning and management function, itself, when required, can convert the discrete tasks of nonprofessionals into skilled-nursing care.

Other situations Medicare recognizes as requiring skilled nursing include those in which a professional or technical person needs to monitor and assess changes in a patient's condition that may require modification of treatment plans, such as postoperative hip fractures or cataract surgery; patients whose physiological problems are complicated by emotional problems, such as depression or anxiety; and patients with a range of clinical needs, such as those who require intravenous feedings, catheterization procedures, and extensive treatment of skin disorders.

States frequently develop their own classification system and definitions for nursing homes. The example presented below is from Massachusetts, where the system is similar to that of many other states and where nursing homes are classified into four levels, each level representing a different type of service with varying staffing requirements. In Massachusetts, Levels I and II are both considered skilled nursing, Level III is classified as intermediate care, and Level IV is the residential-care facility. Below are the state's definitions for each:

(*Level I*) *Intensive Nursing and Rehabilitative Care Facility* shall mean a facility or units thereof that provide continuous skilled-nursing care and an organized program of restorative services in addition to the minimum basic care and services required in these rules and regulations.

(*Level II*) *Skilled-Nursing Care Facility* shall mean a facility or units thereof that provide continuous skilled-nursing care and meaningful availability of restorative services and other therapeutic services in addition to the minimum basic care and services required in these rules and regulations for patients who show potential for improvement or restoration to a stabilized condition or who have a deteriorating condition requiring skilled care.

(*Level III*) *Supportive Nursing Care Facility* shall mean a facility or units thereof that provide routine nursing services and periodic availability of skilled nursing, restorative and other therapeutic services in addition to the minimum basic care and services required in these rules and regulations for patients whose condition is stabilized to the point that they need only supportive care, supervision, and observation.

(*Level IV*) *Residential Care Facility* shall mean a facility or units thereof that provide or arrange to provide in addition to the minimum basic care and services required in these rules and regulations, a supervised supportive and protective living environment and support services for elderly ambulatory residents 50 years of age or older having difficulty in caring for themselves who do not require Level I/II or III nursing care or other medically related services on a routine basis. This facility's services seek to foster personal well-being, independence, an optimal level of psychological functioning, and integration of residents into community living.

While the definitions of the various levels are ambiguous, the states also issue detailed regulations about requirements in terms of specific services and staffing for each level. Illustrative of this is Massachusetts, where, as elsewhere, the newly admitted resident must have a complete physical and medical evaluation, which can be performed by a physician, physician assistant, or nurse practitioner. Time limits on when the patient must have the exam and evaluation vary by skill level; for Level I and Level II admittees, the exam and the medical care plan for the resident must be done within the time zone of five days prior to admission or forty-eight hours after admission. For the Level III and IV residents, who presumably are in a less medically needy situation, the plan's time frame ranges from fourteen days prior to admission to seventy-two hours after admission.

ORGANIZATIONAL BASICS:
Nursing-Home Ownership and Management

Of the 20,000 nursing homes in the United States, approximately 15,000 are owned by individual or corporate private entrepreneurs who operate these facilities as for-profit businesses. About 40 percent of these for-profit homes are owned by chains, while the others usually are family-owned and managed operations. The giant among the publicly owned and traded chains is the California–based Beverly Enterprises, which operates more than 1,000 facilities in forty-six states. Others include the Tacoma, Washington–based Hillhaven Corporation, with close to 400 nursing homes in forty states; Dallas's National Heritage, with 231 homes in twenty-nine states; and the Silver Spring, Maryland–based Manor Care, with 142 homes in twenty-four states. Among the privately held giants are Houston's ARA Living Centers, with 255 homes in thirteen states, and the Milwaukee–based Unicare Health Facilities, with 139 homes in seventeen states. In addition to the large chains, numerous small chains operate several facilities within a state or region.

About 1,000 nursing homes are owned by governmental agencies. For example, my community (Northampton, Massachusetts) has a fifty-bed facility owned by the Veterans Administration and a 120-bed skilled- and intermediate-care nursing home owned by the county government. The latter facility has residents whose bills are paid both privately and by Medicaid.

The third category of ownership, which accounts for approximately 4,000 facilities, is the voluntary, not-for-profit home. These homes, which typically have charitable or religious roots, are organized so that no part of the home's net earnings operate to benefit any private shareholders. Various levels of government have struck a bargain with these organizations so that if they act in and for the public good by eschewing the personal (as opposed to organizational) benefits of profit, the organization will be exempt from federal income taxes as well as state and local real estate and sales taxes.

All of this helps the nursing home's residents in a variety of ways. First, the dollars that a home would have to pay in taxes are now freed up to provide for more staff and programs. Second, charitable or religiously rooted not-for-profit homes frequently are involved in extensive fund-raising projects that provide additional sources of revenue. Illustrative of this fund-raising is one home that I visited where the women's club generates close to $30,000 each year at a donor dinner and another group raises in excess of $10,000 at an annual tennis and golf tournament. For the donor to such not-for-profit nursing homes, there are two incentives: giving to a good cause and a tax deduction for the gift. Third, perhaps because of their charitable roots, not-for-profit homes—and to some extent federally owned homes (particularly Veterans Administration nursing facilities)—do an outstanding job in developing vibrant volunteer programs. Active volunteers play an invaluable role in maintaining contact between the resident and the community, and a secondary but real role in augmenting a nursing home's staff. During my visits to nursing homes, I have seen volunteers reading to residents, leading exercise and sing-along groups, helping the frail elderly write letters or even biographies, and taking people out for a snack or a ride (in one case, in a volunteer's Rolls-Royce). Volunteers come in all sizes and ages. Indeed, one of the most touching nursing-home programs I saw was one in which a group of teenagers at a summer camp once a week spent the morning visiting the residents. From a manpower perspective, the tens of thousands of hours that volunteers spend in a nursing home can provide the equivalent of having a large staff.

Another important aspect of the not-for-profit home is the philosophical orientation, which means that the "profits" (i.e., any excess of income over expenses) are to be reinvested in the home. In practice, many not-for-profits do not generate significant profits because they are continuously spending their money on staff or on items that a for-profit home is unlikely to purchase, such as vehicles to transport residents to outside activities.

The clearest manifestation of the differences among the not-for-profit, government, and for-profit facilities is seen in the staffing. National data show that the average number of full-time equivalent employees per 100 beds for proprietary (for-profit) homes was 65.4; for the not-for-profit homes, it was 83.8; and for government homes, 87.6. As I looked at homes, I saw the confirmation of this data on a local basis. The private homes tended to have between 15 and 20 percent fewer staff members than the not-for-profit ones. Although some of this staffing difference occurs in the arguably secondary administrative areas, the greatest part of the difference can be found in the number of nursing and therapeutic service staff in the not-for-profit home.

Finally, the not-for-profit (and to some extent the government-owned) homes have a built-in community watchdog group, usually called the board of directors or the board of trustees. Such a group, frequently comprising prominent citizens, has the responsibility for overseeing the home's operations. Typical of many of the board members whom I have met over the years is James Reich, president of the board of directors of the Riverview Center for Jewish Seniors in Pittsburgh. His work for Riverview is not confined to board meetings and telephone conversations. Indeed, when I made an unannounced visit to Reich at his Squirrel Hill clothing store on a busy Thursday night, he immediately dropped what he was doing, took me into his back office, and proceeded to talk knowledgeably and at length about the Pittsburgh nursing-home scene. The enthusiasm of Jim Reich and thousands of other people around the country who give of themselves to voluntary nursing-home boards gets translated into staffing, programs, and other activities that reverberate to the benefit of residents.

MANAGEMENT BASICS

The day-to-day management of the nursing home is the responsibility of a nursing-home administrator who is licensed by the state. While state requirements for licensure vary, basically they include some combination of education in health-care administration and experience in the field. Subsequently, there usually are continuing-education requirements necessary for relicensure.

In nursing homes, to a far greater degree than in other health-care organizations such as hospitals, management plays a key role. The administrator's job is that of translating the federal and state rules and regulations as well as the policies of the owner or governing body into the operations of the home. I have seen numerous examples of administrators around the country who have made a difference in their nursing homes.

One of my earliest stops was in the St. Louis suburb of Chesterfield, where I visited with Miner Brown, director of the 276-bed Jewish Center for the Aged from 1975 to 1989. In a 1984 *St. Louis Magazine* article, "Moe" Brown, who was then forty-three, was described as energetic and excited about geriatric health care. The writer also noted that "Brown's most extraordinary talent lies in his appreciation of how the environment affects people's well-being." This quite-correct observation has been translated into action in a number of ways by Brown and his successor.

One of the first features that caught my eye outside of the home was a children's playground. When I asked Brown about it, he told me it had cost the home about $4,000, a sum he had had no trouble raising. The playground's purpose was simple: It gives grandchildren and children something to do when they visit the home, and it makes for a more congenial and homelike atmosphere for everyone. The second aspect that attracted my attention was that none of the staff members at the nursing home wore uniforms. As Brown sees it, uniforms are barriers to both relationships and communications.

In his zest for providing a less institutional environment, Brown encouraged numerous programs, such as the use of the thousands of feet of wall space as a rotating art gallery, the development of an active gardening therapy program, and sensory stimulation activities. The gardens also serve as the setting for professional musicians who provide the public Starlight Concerts series as well as for the annual Festival of Ages, a one-day crafts show with a carnival and barbecue. While a number of aspects of the Chesterfield home impressed me, there was a small dining program—called "Specialty of the House"—that I found simple and innovative: For a modest fee, residents can host small, private candlelight dinner parties for friends and family at the nursing home.

In Seattle, Washington, at the Caroline Kline Galland Home, the director, Joshua Gortler, is making a crucial difference in the lives of the home's 145 residents, half of whom are Medicaid recipients. For example, Gortler—whose background is in social work—had all the nursing stations cut down to knee height so that residents in wheelchairs would be at the same level as the nurses. In response to the personal needs of the residents for independence, nourishment, and socialization, he had instituted twenty-four-hour minisnack bars at each unit, with juice machines and a small refrigerator stocked daily with healthful snacks. To respond to the residents' emotional needs, Gortler has retained an experienced psychiatrist who comes into the home each week to provide training for staff as well as consultations for residents. As I walked through the home, I saw many examples of how Gortler, like Moe Brown, is sensitive to the way physical surroundings affect residents. This sensitivity manifests itself in the colors used in the home, the three or four different styles of furniture bought by the home so that residents could select the bed or dresser they wanted in their rooms, and the artwork in the halls and dining areas. In addition, the home has a dog named Erin, who wanders the halls, providing an opportunity for the residents to relax by petting a gentle animal.

While in Seattle, I also visited the 150-bed Seattle Keiro Home, which opened in 1987 as a facility for the elderly Japanese community in the Pacific Northwest. Although the administrator was not there, I met with his deputy, Anne Arakaki-Lock, and saw how their attitudes, as well as those of the community, affected that home. From the moment I entered the grounds of the home, with its traditional Japanese gardens and shrine-type entryway, I felt its sensitivity to the residents. The signs throughout the home were in Japanese and English, and in the therapy rooms were large cue cards for staff with the various essential words in Japanese and English. Activities included videotaped Japanese television programs and ikebana (flower-arranging) sessions. During the noon meal, I observed fresh flowers on each table in the dining hall, quiet music being played by an organist, and a menu that offered traditional Japanese foods about half the time. On the floors, the monotony of the hallways is broken up by a number of tokonomas—alcoves with hanging scrolls and traditional vases of flowers. The home's name, *Keiro*, means "respected elder," and it certainly lived up to its name.

Three thousand miles away, in Portland, Maine, I visited with Ron Tardiff at the 200-bed St. Joseph's Manor. My tour of St. Joseph's began in the front lobby, where there was a large photomural of Portland's famous lighthouse. Tardiff explained that this had not been placed there merely to decorate the wall but rather to help residents, particularly new ones, find a point of identification with the home and the Portland environment. To the greatest extent possible, Tardiff, like many of the other administrators I met, tries to keep the residents involved in the communities outside the nursing home. In the case of St. Joseph's, this involves picnics, bus trips to a local lobster restaurant, shopping trips to the Maine Mall, and occasionally outside performances by resident groups such as the SJM Singers.

Elsewhere in New England, I met with Larry Knowles, administrator of the Vernon Advent Christian Home in Vernon, Vermont, a complex that includes independent living units, retirement apartments, and a fifty-nine-bed nursing home. Knowles, who lives on the grounds of the facility and certainly puts in far more than forty hours a week, is similar to many people associated with religious-affiliated homes in that he sees his job as a type of religious calling. When I visited with him in the summer of 1988, he told me about an award the home had just received from the Vermont Council on Aging for maintaining a facility where 99 percent of the residents are free from chemical and mechanical restraints. In explaining the program, he gave credit to the director of nursing, who initially questioned the supposition that restraints were necessary.

On one of my swings through the South, I visited the 120-bed Jewish Home in Atlanta, where I met with Mark Ponder, the director of Health Services, and learned of an extraordinary program instituted by Ponder and his administrator, Deborah Beards. Every weekday morning, all of the home's department heads spend a half hour helping the nursing staff on the residential floors. The help these executives provide changes from day to day but may include assisting in the feeding, dressing, or transporting of residents. Sometimes, it involves merely sitting and talking with someone for a few moments. If this innovative program works, the home's entire management team will have a continuing and clearer picture of what is going on with the home's residents.

Finally, I am reminded of an incident that occurred on a warm summer evening a few years ago in the lobby of the 200-bed Jewish Nursing Home of Western Massachusetts. It was about 6:00 P.M., and Howard Braverman, the home's newly appointed director, was heading through the lobby to take a walk before a 6:30 P.M. board dinner scheduled for the auditorium. As he was leaving, the home's security guard called after him and asked whether the snack bar should be kept closed that night. Not comprehending the question, Braverman asked the guard what he meant. The guard, a gentle but bearlike cigar-chewing veteran of countless years at the home, said that it had been the policy to close the snack bar when the adjacent auditorium was used for such events as board or auxiliary meetings. Apparently the sight of the elderly in wheelchairs or using walkers was discomforting for some visitors. With obvious annoyance, Braverman replied, "Open the snack bar. This is the residents' home, not ours. We are the intruders!"

While these examples illustrate the important role that management plays in the quality of life for nursing-home residents, the people with whom residents have the most direct and often most crucial contact are the members of the medical and nursing staffs.

MEDICAL-STAFF BASICS

Speak to anyone associated with nursing homes and they will tell you the same thing: "The residents are coming to us in a more debilitated state of health; they are older and need more intense care." From this should flow the conclusion that nursing homes have a significant medical staff—that is, a physician—present. Unfortunately, that is simply not the case.

While all nursing homes have physicians designated as medical directors, the reality is that most homes rarely have the benefit of a significant medical presence beyond the state-mandated minimum, which in some cases is as low as four hours per month. Typically, the medical director spends a few hours at the home each week, rapidly checking on a number of residents and spending even less time on the paperwork of medical care.

Each resident normally is required to have an attending physician in addition to the medical director—whose job is primarily the administrative overview of the medical care at the home. In many cases the attending doctor also is the medical director, but residents retain the right to select their own physicians. So, if it is mutually acceptable, the family physician may continue to serve as the nursing-home resident's attending physician.

Admission to nursing homes requires a physician's order, although sometimes a nurse practitioner can provide an admission order, which then is countersigned by a physician.

An exceptionally well-run home will have a full-time medical director who is a gerontologist—a physician whose clinical training as well as personal commitment is in the care of the elderly. Such a person is most likely to be knowledgeable about those clinical issues of geriatric care that have an impact on the daily life of a resident. For example, there is considerable literature about medication problems with the elderly, a situation that a full-time medical director would no doubt be aware of and interested in evaluating. Some recent literature suggests that as many as half of the frail elderly who have been classified as totally incontinent can become continent through careful evaluation of their type of problem (e.g., urge, reflex, stress, overflow, etc.) and appropriate medical intervention. A physician working full time with a group of people facing these problems on a daily basis is more likely to be attuned to resolving these issues than the occasional visiting physician whose nursing-home rounds take five minutes per resident.

The full-time medical director, typically found in the not-for-profit or government home (particularly facilities associated with medical schools and other training programs), is exactly as the term implies—full time. One simple question will easily determine the status of any home's medical staffing: How many hours per week does the medical director spend at the home?

While the ideal model of the full-time medical director does indeed exist in many homes, there are several other options that homes can utilize in order to meet the need for a full-time committed medical presence. A 120-bed home in Florida, for example, employs a twenty-hour-per-week medical director but provides him with an office so he can conduct his private practice on the premises, thus ensuring his availability for emergencies and unusual problems. A number of nursing homes' staffs consist of several physicians whose total hours at the home exceed forty but who split their time between appointments at the home and teaching at a medical school. One home I visited employs a team of five physicians, each of whom takes responsibility for a different day of the week. Together they form a group practice for the home's residents. At Shalom Geriatric Center in Kansas City, Missouri, six to eight senior medical students are at the home three times per week, augmenting the services of the part-time medical director and a full-time physician who is supported by a gerontology medical fellowship from the University of Kansas Medical Center.

Another option that also has merit is the combination of a part-time medical director and a full-time geriatric nurse practitioner who is a registered nurse with advanced training in assessing and treating the needs of the elderly. At these homes where such an arrangement has been developed, the geriatric nurse practitioners function under the supervision of a physician; through the use of standard clinical protocols, they are able to diagnose and treat a significant percentage of the primary-care needs of a nursing home's population.

NURSING-STAFF BASICS

Central to the staffing of any long-term-care facility is nursing, which usually represents about 60 percent of the total employee complement. Three distinct groups of people provide the care delivered by the nursing department: registered nurses, licensed practical (or vocational) nurses, and aides.

Registered nurses (RNs) are those who have completed the requirements of a two-year community-college program, a three-year hospital-based nursing school, or a four-year college-based nursing program. Following these programs, the graduate takes a state licensing exam, and, if successful, is entitled to the designation RN, or registered nurse. In terms of practice, the RN has the greatest level of responsibility and authority for delivering care to a resident, which normally includes technical tasks such as giving medications and inserting and removing catheters, and supervisory and managerial functions such as developing a nursing treatment plan for a resident and ensuring that the plan is implemented.

At the next level are the licensed practical (or vocational) nurses (LPNs or LVNs), who, on average, account for between 15 and 20 percent of the total nursing staff. In functional terms, much of what the LPN does overlaps with the work of the RN, but the supervisory responsibility remains with the registered nurse. It is common to see LPNs taking vital signs (temperature, blood pressure, and respiration); administering medications; giving enemas; monitoring intravenous fluids; and in some cases supervising the nursing activities of a unit. The educational requirements for licensed practical or vocational nurses vary from state to state but in general they include passing a state licensure exam subsequent to either graduation from a vocational high school program or a one-year post–high school training program.

The third and most populous group is the aides, who make up almost 70 percent of the nursing staff. Under current state and federal regulations, aides must receive between eighty and a hundred hours of training before certification. Aides are central to the delivery of a range of day-to-day care. For example, they are the people who bathe, dress, feed, and transport the residents.

Of greatest importance to anyone looking for a nursing home is knowing how the regulations differentiate the required nursing times for the different levels of residents. The crucial measure used is "hours of nursing care per resident per day." In my travels, I have found that 90 percent of the nursing-home administrators or nursing directors could give me an instant answer to the question: "How many nursing hours per resident per day do you have?" In several instances, I did the arithmetic myself after the administrator provided me with the raw data. For example, in one 88-bed home, the administrator supplied a figure of 1,848 as the total weekly nursing hours. This, divided by 616 (seven days times the number of residents), produced a figure of three hours of nursing care per resident per day.

Each state sets minimum hours per resident per day by level of care. There are several ways to find out these minimums, but the easiest is to check with the administrator of a local nursing home. A second way is to call the state agency responsible for regulating nursing homes—the state department of health usually is a good place to start. A third—and interesting—way is to read the regulations yourself; these usually are available in the law library at the county courthouse or a local law school. The regulations will provide the essential rules of thumb necessary for understanding what you will be evaluating. For example, Massachusetts regulations require that Level I facilities provide, in addition to adequate management and supervisory level nurses, 2.6 hours of nursing care per resident per day (of which 0.6 hour must be provided by either registered nurses or licensed practical or licensed vocational nurses). The remaining two hours of care normally are provided by an aide, who typically has had about two and a half weeks of training. The Level II requirement is for a total of two hours of nursing time per resident per day, with aides providing 1.4 hours and registered or licensed nurses 0.6 hour. Finally, the Level III requirement is a total of 1.4 hours, with aides providing one hour and the professional staff 0.4 hour.

What I have seen in practice is that the good nursing homes rarely go below the three-hour rate and frequently are close to 3.5 hours per resident per day. The extra half hour per day may not sound like much, but it does result in significant variations among facilities. For example, it could make the difference between a hectic or a relaxed environment or an enthusiastic or a burned-out staff. On a very practical level, it could spell the difference between having sufficient staff and expecting families to provide regular assistance or employ nurses or sitters for the residents.

SOCIAL-SERVICES BASICS

For many families, the first contact with a nursing home is through its social-services department. In promotional literature and residents' handbooks, this department frequently is defined as being either responsible for the emotional and social needs of residents or, as Atlanta's A. G. Rhodes Home states, ". . . as a liaison between the resident and staff of the home"— sort of an internal ombudsman. In practice, this means that the social-services staff usually provides information about the home and its services and the cost of care or help in applying for financial assistance. If a decision is made to apply to a home, social workers usually process the applications and may be involved in the testing and evaluation of the applicant. On the day of admission, someone from social services commonly is responsible for squiring a person through the transition from home to institution. The social-services staff also deals with any problems that arise during this period—such as displeasure with a room or roommate or difficulties with the nursing home's schedule. Social services are required for nursing-home licensure, so states set educational requirements for social workers and stipulate the number of social-work hours a nursing home must offer. Typically, the smaller the home, the fewer the hours that must be offered.

While I have met some social-services people who appeared to be merely marketing operatives with a primary function of recruiting financially secure private-pay residents, most of those I encountered were more interested in helping people than in filling beds. Harvey Shankman, director of social services at the 334-bed Menorah Park in Beechwood, Ohio, is an example of such a professional. His basic attitude is: ". . . We are not looking for business." What this means is that his job as well as that of his staff of four is to educate families about themselves, their needs, and the other resources that are available in the community to serve these needs.

Following admission, the social worker frequently takes on the job of case manager, thus becoming an in-house liaison and ombudsman for the resident. This task involves resolving adjustment problems for both the resident and the family and responding to the needs of staff vis-à-vis a resident. For example, the nursing staff may want to have a resident or a resident's family clarify instructions concerning resuscitation of the resident in case of cardiac arrest.

THERAPEUTIC-SERVICES BASICS

Therapeutic services is a broad category that includes physical, occupational, speech, art, music, and pet therapy, as well as several other specialized services. Despite the importance of these various therapies in maintaining and possibly restoring a person's health, the requirements imposed upon nursing homes for providing such services are limited. For example, the Massachusetts regulations, which label therapeutic services as restorative therapy, provide a model of ambiguity when they note that Level II facilities "shall provide meaningful availability of restorative therapy services beyond restorative and maintenance nursing care."

The two most commonly available therapeutic services are

physical and occupational therapy. The focus of physical therapy is the restoration of function, prevention of disability, and relief of pain. In response to a physician's order, the physical therapist develops a treatment plan as well as an evaluation that includes tests of muscle strength, gait analysis, body-part measurements, and a range of motion assessment. Treatments typically used by a physical-therapy department include whirlpools, ultrasound, hot packs, massage, parallel bars, and a variety of muscle-building devices, such as wall pulleys.

Occupational therapy is not "job training," but rather a significant component of the physical and emotional rehabilitation process. Occupational therapy concentrates on channeling the strength developed in physical therapy into daily living activities, such as homemaking skills and manual arts and crafts. Some occupational-therapy departments are involved in the design of an extraordinary variety of splints and other gadgets for assisting residents in regaining their independence.

Programs in art, music, and pet therapy, found in some homes, should be distinguished from recreational activities that involve arts and crafts, music, or pets. To point up this distinction, we can contrast what goes on at the 192-bed Shalom Geriatric Center in Kansas City with what happens in most nursing homes. The first difference is that Shalom employs the equivalent of almost two full-time art therapists. They are primarily therapists whose job is to help residents use art as a vehicle for expressing their emotions. At Shalom, the art therapists evaluate each incoming resident, prepare notes for the resident's charts, and utilize the resident's projects as input for psychiatric evaluations. At a more typical home, art is merely a recreational activity run by volunteers whose function is to help residents create; these volunteers do not provide any input for the therapeutic programs. Music, dance, pet, and several other therapies are similar to art therapy in the sense that if they exist in a home, it usually is as a recreational activity without a therapeutic dimension— although in rare cases, as at Shalom, the commitment is made to utilize these modalities for therapeutic purposes.

There is a broad spectrum of ways nursing homes organize the delivery of therapeutic services. In the best of situations, such as at Golden Acres, a 265-bed home in Dallas, the home employs a full-time staff, which usually includes physical and occupational therapists and aides as well as individuals trained in the expressive therapies. Such a commitment involves not only the cost of staffing a department (eight people, for instance, at Golden Acres) but also the cost of building and maintaining a 4,000-square-foot facility with an inventory of expensive equipment ranging from whirlpools to kilns.

In general, state regulations require only that nursing homes have services available to residents and that the services be provided on the written orders of a physician. In practice, the concept of availability means that the facilities contract for services on an "as-needed" basis. In many homes, residents do not receive physical or occupational therapy on a regular schedule but only get the service for short-term needs from contract physical or occupational therapists. Unfortunately, too many nursing homes have no dedicated area for such therapies and the space utilized is often minimal and unpleasant.

ACTIVITIES AND RECREATION BASICS

Although all nursing homes have some type of activities program, here again there are great variations. Since most state and federal requirements are ambiguous and rather minimal, the differences are a function of a home's resources and its commitment to an activities program that is functionally related to the general therapy program.

A typical small home with 100 to 125 beds may have one or two full-time activities staff members with training that varies from on-the-job experience to college degrees in recreational therapy. In terms of programs, virtually every nursing home has some of the following activities: arts and crafts, exercise, current-events discussions, games, religious services, and the old standby, bingo. What distinguishes the run-of-the-mill place from the particularly interesting facility is the quality of the staff planning and organizing that goes into delivering a wide variety of timely offerings. For example, some homes give lip service to the residents' need for a library (and in some cases, the state requirement for one) merely by having a shelf full of discarded books and magazines recycled from a dentist's office. Others have fully stocked libraries with large-print books, image intensifiers (magnifying glasses), and even books written in the mother tongues of the residents.

One activity that several homes have developed is a sheltered workshop in which residents can spend several hours each day doing basic manual-labor jobs for pay.

The Fairfield Jewish Home in Fairfield, Connecticut, has a particularly interesting program in which they offer residents an annual four-day camping trip and an overnight trip to a resort hotel. Both of these excursions require an amazing amount of organization and dedication, since they involve transporting, housing, and feeding a busload of residents, nurses, and ancillary staff, as well as continual overseeing of the health and well-being of the residents. Obviously, it would be much easier not to have such a program, but Dennis Magid, the home's director, points out that such programs are of immense psychological importance because they allow the participants to feel less isolated from the rest of the world. The programs also offer the nonparticipants something special to look forward to at some future date.

DIETARY BASICS

After eating hundreds of meals in nursing homes and thousands in hospitals, I think it is fair to say that institutional food is not a substitute for "home cooking." Eating at a nursing home, even in the best of places, is problematic. The atmosphere of a small or large dining hall, the restrictions on diet, and the strictures on time grate on everyone. Indeed, if we were forced to eat all our meals in the same dining room of the same hotel 365 times a year, it also would become tiresome.

State and federal regulations on food service fit into the usual pattern of lofty objectives and ambiguous standards. A full-time dietitian—or, as in most cases, a consulting dietitian—has the responsibility of overseeing the nutritional content of meals as well as the diets of individual residents. Typically, a physician will order a special diet, such as low cholesterol, and the dietitian reviews the diet and ensures that it is adequate in all other aspects (that is, calorically and nutritionally). The actual dietary operation is run by a food-service manager, who may or may not be a dietitian. As in all other areas, there are significant differences in how meals are planned, prepared, and delivered. It is easy to envision, for example, looking forward to meals at the Seattle Keiro Home and a number of other facilities. On the other hand, there are a great many homes that, while providing nutritionally adequate meals, do so in dining halls that minutes earlier were dayrooms and usually are rather reminiscent of army mess halls.

THE REST OF THE HOME

Dozens of other people are involved in the smooth operation of a good-quality nursing home: Laundry workers tend to the institution's laundry as well as the personal clothing of the residents; maintenance workers ensure the safety and mechanical functioning of the facility; the crucial housekeeping staff keeps the place presentable and inoffensive; and business-office people order supplies, pay bills, bill residents, and may act as personal bankers for residents. All of these people—along with the nurses, technicians, and others—act as the surrogate family for the residents. Their caring attitudes and behavior make all the difference between a home that is supportive and rewarding and one that offers a horrible, distasteful, and degrading experience.

HOSPITALS AND NURSING HOMES

While most of us wish to avoid hospitals, we recognize that at some point in life there is a good chance we might spend a few days in one for some reason or another. In general, the visit is short and, thanks to the new systems of reimbursement, getting shorter. Our expectation is that the hospital experience will be "high tech, low touch"; that is, we will be poked and probed and treated with a full range of drugs and other therapy. We do not expect to develop long-term personal relationships with nurses, therapists, aides, housekeepers, food-service employees, or the administrator. The whole process, in fact, is expected to be impersonal, albeit friendly. In the end, we will have a repaired body and will return to our previous activities with a few modifications. Sort of a "Jiffy Lube" experience for the body.

Nursing homes are not hospitals. Quite the contrary! Because of the problems with which they deal and the nature of the clientele they serve, nursing homes tend to be "low tech, high touch" institutions. What a person did for himself or herself in the past is now done with the assistance of others. The nurses and aides help the elderly person get out of bed in the morning, go to the toilet, bathe, dress, eat, and take medication. The activities staff is around all day helping to stimulate the person's interest in and zest for life; the food-service personnel are cooking for the resident's health and enjoyment; the therapists are busily fighting the uphill battle against a deteriorating body (and perhaps mind); and the social-services staff is trying to solve problems that range from financing the care to unpleasant roommates.

De facto, the nursing home is a new and often permanent place to live, and to a significant extent, the staff becomes an extended family. Staff members must take care of the intimate details of the resident's life and, in the end, they often can be seen sitting next to an elderly resident and holding a hand as life quietly slips away.

A number of years ago, the president of the board of directors of an excellent nursing home told me that because a nursing home is never "home," even in the best of situations, he did not think anyone should move into a nursing home unless it was "absolutely necessary." Unfortunately, the concept of "absolutely necessary" is ambiguous. In the next chapter, I shall address this central question of the need for moving into a nursing home.

TWO

THE NEED FOR A NURSING HOME

I couldn't take care of my apartment.... I needed care.

—Mrs. G. K., ninety-year-old nursing-home resident,
Cleveland, Ohio

A few years ago, while on a trip to South Florida, I stopped in to see Bill Goodman, an eighty-three-year-old man who was dying of cancer. The visit took place in the comfortable, one-bedroom condominium that he shared with Mildred, his seventy-eight-year-old spouse, who herself had health problems that included a recent heart attack and a stroke.

By all accounts, Bill Goodman was a perfect candidate for a nursing home, since he needed assistance in eating, bathing, dressing, using the toilet, and transferring from a bed to a chair or out of the chair and into a bed. However, despite his dependent state, he was able to stay home because of Mildred's support, the aid of a local hospice worker who came in twice a week to bathe him, and their fortunate economic status, which allowed them to have nursing assistance around the clock.

The Goodman case illustrates the important point that "need for nursing-home care" can be assessed objectively, but the fact that a need exists does not necessarily mean that someone has to move to a nursing home. Why and how did Bill avoid that? There are several reasons. First, like most people, he did not want to end his life in a nursing home. He wanted to spend as much of his time as possible in the familiar surroundings of his own home. Second, he had the support of Mildred, which translated into a willingness to radically alter

23

her lifestyle to accommodate Bill's nursing needs. For example, not everyone would be so generous in allowing an unknown nurse's aide to move into their apartment and share their bedroom. Third, he had the financial resources to pay almost three full-time salaries for round-the-clock care.

The Goodmans were also fortunate to find competent and willing nursing assistants. Indeed, he was lucky to have located his caregivers just as they were completing another long-term nursing engagement. Sometimes, nursing assistance simply is not available, and the family is unable to provide the necessary care. For example, a few years ago I received a letter from a colleague saying he was taking early retirement to spend more time with his wife, who was being institutionalized because of Alzheimer's disease. For years she had been taken care of at home by a rotating army of nurses, but finally he had exhausted all the noninstitutional resources in the community and the only remaining option was a nursing home.

Bill Goodman also was lucky to have a physician who was supportive of his desire to stay at home and willing to work to accommodate those needs. Finally, Bill and Mildred had the good fortune to live in a community that had such resources as the hospice to provide the essential backup to the family and other caregivers.

Not everyone who wishes to do so can avoid a nursing home—and in many instances a nursing home is a much better place to be than one's own home. In the following sections of this chapter, I shall examine the need for nursing-home care from the perspectives of residents, families, physicians, and bureaucrats.

THE RESIDENTS' PERSPECTIVE

Traveling throughout the country, I interviewed scores of elderly nursing-home residents. One of my routine questions was: Why are you in a nursing home? The most common answer—whether they had come from a hospital or from a private residence—was that they needed a level of care and supervision that only a nursing home was prepared to deliver. And frequently, some type of especially traumatic event, such as a death or a serious illness, precipitated admission to the nursing home. Here are some of their voices:

I was in shock after my husband died. I was hospitalized, overmedicated, misdiagnosed as having Alzheimer's disease when it was the drugs that were confusing me.
                                    —*Mrs. I. M., seventy-seven years old*

I came here because I lost my family and my health.
                                    —*Mrs. E. W., eighty-three years old*

I took sick, my wife died, and my doctor recommended a nursing home.
                                    —*Mr. M. R., ninety-four years old*

I was in a bad depression after I lost a daughter. I wasn't eating.
                                    —*Mrs. S. W., ninety years old*

Finally, many of these people were also logistically alone in the world. For example, they were people who never married or were now widows or widowers; they had no children or their children lived in distant communities or lived distant lives in local communities. Sometimes, the elderly simply did not want to disrupt the lives of their families, and they viewed a nursing home as the best available option:

My husband was here for 1½ years and I sort of got tired traveling every day to visit him, so I decided to join him in the home. After six months he passed away and I stayed on.
                                    —*Mrs. G. S., eighty-six years old*

When my wife passed away, I did not want to live with my children. I told them they have their own lives . . . why should I go mess them up.
                                    —*Mr. S. R., ninety-one years old*

I didn't want to go live with my children; it isn't a good idea. It's nice, but it is not a home of my own.
                                    —*Mr. M. R., ninety-six years old*

I surely wouldn't want to live in a home with my children; they have different ideas.
                                    —*Mrs. S. W., ninety years old*

*I lived with my son for eight months and then by mutual agreement,
I came here.*
                    —*Mrs. I. M., seventy-seven years old*

I was living with my daughter and I did not like living with her.
                    —*Mrs. S. D., eighty-four years old*

*When I was ninety-one, my wife got very sick and moved into the
nursing home. I came with her, and after she died I just stayed on.*
                    —*Mr. S. C., ninety-six years old*

My children are not interested in me.
                    —*Mrs. G. F., eighty-seven years old*

The testimony of these residents demonstrates that the concept of "need" for nursing-home care is multidimensional. For
some, "need" means the home can satisfy some medical or
clinical requirements—that is, the home functions as something akin to a sub-acute hospital. For others, and perhaps the
majority of residents, the home is the apparent answer to
complex psychological and social problems ranging from the
inability to secure adequate household and personal-care assistance to familial estrangement. Sometimes it is simply a
place where there are people with whom to interact all day. In
the next section, I will examine "need" from the perspective of
those who frequently are responsible for the decision and often carry heavy burdens of guilt about "putting" someone in a
nursing home.

THE FAMILY'S PERSPECTIVE

A family's perspective on the need for a nursing home frequently is of crucial importance to the final decision to insti-
tutionalize one of its members. Generally the family is dealing
with one of three situations: In the first type of situation, the
family member requires short-stay post-hospital care for rehabilitation or skilled nursing. In this instance, the nursing
home is functioning as a sub-acute hospital and there is no

intent to keep the patient more than a few weeks or months. The decision about institutionalizing such a person is fairly easy, since the only true alternative is continued hospitalization.

A variation of this type of situation occurs when the family member is going to a nursing home after a hospitalization and there is no intention of having that person move back into a private residence. In a sense, the hospitalization presents the opportunity for a family to move an elderly person out of their home and essentially trap him or her in a nursing home when the patient is most vulnerable. In one family where I saw this occur, the nursing-home resident was bitter over the "ambush" until the day he died, and he took every opportunity to share his bitterness with his children.

The second type of situation and the third—where a person moves directly from home to a nursing home—are actually quite analogous, because they bring up a variety of conflicting feelings for the family. These feelings range from a sense of perceived duty—"We have to do this in the best interests of the family or family member"—to a strong sense of guilt and betrayal—"We should have been able to care for Mom." On the following pages are three case studies that illustrate the issues and problems families face in dealing with the second and third types of situations.

CASE 1: The Williams Family

I first met Mrs. Williams several years ago when she attended a lecture I presented to the residents of a large geriatric center. She was a well-dressed and attractive woman who I later learned was fifty-eight years old. She listened attentively, and because she was sitting next to a gray-haired woman with whom she had walked in, I assumed she was the woman's daughter. As my presentation moved into the discussion phase, I decided to engage people by asking questions. So I began questioning some of the center's residents and then moved on to some guests, Mrs. Williams among them. When I asked her a question, she smiled politely and said, "Hello." I then moved closer to her, asked the question again, and received the same response. After the lecture, I learned that she was a participant in the center's adult day-care program and was a victim of Alzheimer's disease.

About a year after I met Mrs. Williams, she was admitted to a nursing home. Several months after that, I had a chance to talk with her sixty-one-year-old husband, who shared with me the situation that the family had faced:

> For the past three years, I have been running a nursing home in my house. I even had a hospital bed there and housekeeping and nursing staff twenty-four hours a day. I needed someone there to watch my wife all the time. Even though she looked well, she needed help with everything, including eating. And she could not communicate. Friends drifted away; if they only knew the importance of a kiss or touch.
>
> I was never able to take care of everything. There was a parade of staff and I had to help schedule things among three people. Sometimes she needed an enema and the staff had trouble giving it to her; the aides were sometimes not qualified. I would come home from work at 4 o'clock and spend half an hour coaxing my wife to go to the toilet. I would just sit there and hold her hand. She also fell a few times and it was difficult to get her off the floor.
>
> Even though the day-care center was good, it wasn't enough. The whole family was being victimized by this disease. I wound up going to a psychiatrist. The final straw was I couldn't work, couldn't do my job. She had fallen down again and I had to get the ambulance over to pick her up. I wanted her to have both activity and dignity.
>
> Putting her in the nursing home was an emotional defeat. But it is the best place for her. There are competent staff around all day and I visit all the time. My kids and I are trying to get back to our lives now.

CASE 2: The Brown Family

In the space of fifteen months, the four children in the Brown family had to deal with the trauma of placing both their mother and their father in a nursing home. The case of the eighty-four-year-old Mr. Brown was in many ways the easier. During the eighteen months preceding his institutionalization in a skilled-nursing facility, he had suffered three strokes, and although his eighty-year-old wife had tried to care for him after the first two strokes, the burden after the third stroke was overwhelming. With some assistance from their physician, the family was able to place Mr. Brown in a facility about two miles from their home.

Shortly after Mr. Brown moved into the nursing home, the youngest of their children, Anita, a thirty-seven-year-old part-time commercial artist, gave up her apartment and moved home, ostensibly to care for her mother. As it turned out, Anita kept an irregular schedule so there still was a need for someone to provide assistance to Mrs. Brown, who suffered from depression as well as Parkinson's disease.

The other three children, all of whom had families and lived between one and three hours away from their mother, became increasingly concerned about her welfare. After a seemingly endless series of long-distance phone calls, it was suggested that Mrs. Brown get some part-time help. Anita vetoed the idea, stating that she had moved home "to take care of Mom."

Finally, three months before my meeting with Bernard Brown, the eldest son, a crisis occurred when Mrs. Brown wandered into the emergency room of the local hospital and was admitted for psychiatric observation. This hospitalization brought all the children together to confer. It was clear to all but Anita that something had to be done. What the family arranged was continued hospitalization in a private institution that would accept their mother for a short stay. While the results of this institutionalization were positive, there was still no long-term resolution of Mrs. Brown's situation.

The next step was to arrange for twenty-four-hour care by aides and housekeeping staff. This approach was satisfactory for approximately a month, but then the first group of staff left and the family and their mother had to contend with a parade of unskilled employees.

After that, the family tried to get Mrs. Brown into the same facility as her husband, but because she was a Level II or perhaps III person, and Mr. Brown's home was primarily Level I, she was not able to get in. Finally, the children arranged for her to move into a not-for-profit home about fifteen miles from Bernard's house. They hoped that this facility would offer more social contact for Mrs. Brown as well as provide her with the kind of assistance she was not receiving at home.

In general, Mrs. Brown has prospered in her new environment, the family is relieved that she is being properly taken care of, and the three older children are pleased they no longer have to deal with Anita about caring for their mother. Furthermore, preparations are now under way for transferring Mr. Brown so he will be in the same home as Mrs. Brown.

CASE 3: The Lincoln Family

For thirteen years after Dr. John Lincoln retired from his professorship at the local university, he kept himself busy with his hobbies of stamp collecting, reading, and gardening, plus his duties as a volunteer at the local hospital. Toward the end of this period, arthritis in his hips and lower back began to make mobility increasingly difficult and painful.

At the urging of his oldest child, a pediatrician, Dr. Lincoln entered the hospital and had a bilateral hip replacement. After the operation, Dr. Lincoln worked very hard at the various prescribed exercises and physical therapy, but the deterioration of his back and the pain in the hip made for difficult days and nights.

His wife, Pat, who still worked twenty hours per week in a local insurance office, was a devoted helpmate during the entire period. She always got up early to get him set for the morning. She would help him get out of bed and make the trip to the toilet. After that, she would help him dress for the day and prepare his breakfast and lunch. In the afternoon and evening, she would again help him with his toileting and then prepare supper. Later she would help him get ready for bed. Twice a week, a home-health-care agency would send an aide to the home to help bathe Dr. Lincoln. Several times a week, the Lincoln children would stop by and provide some relief for their mother and company for their father. Once or twice a month, the family would help Dr. Lincoln into a wheelchair and take him for a ride or a trip to church. This pattern went on for over a year until Mrs. Lincoln's health gave out and she needed hospitalization for lower back pain—a condition doubtless related to the work this five-foot-tall woman undertook in maneuvering her 200-pound husband around their home.

Mrs. Lincoln's hospitalization clarified the need for the family to enlist additional help. The oldest child was able to make arrangements for a person to go in forty hours a week to aid her parents with cooking, cleaning, and minor aide duties. However, a physical and psychological burden still rested on Mrs. Lincoln. Finally, after another two months, the oldest child's husband called a family meeting and stated: "In everybody's best interest, Pop needs to be in a nursing home." Everyone agreed that he was right, but the next problem was deciding who was going to tell Dr. Lincoln. Mrs. Lincoln said time and again that she could not do it. It was not until months after Dr. Lincoln's institutionalization that she was able to acknowledge her acute sense of guilt and failure over his admission. She said she felt she had betrayed her husband. The youngest child, himself a thirty-year-old lawyer, was hesitant. The daughter stepped forward and volunteered. What she recalls most vividly about telling her father was that he already knew it was something that had to be done.

In these three cases, despite the availability of financial resources and the best efforts of a supportive family, it became necessary for someone to move into a nursing home. In each instance the move came after a period of at-home care that was marked by increasing emotional frustration and physical debilitation. The move into the nursing home, while traumatic, signaled the beginning of a new and more organized relationship within the family units.

THE PHYSICIAN'S PERSPECTIVE

Nursing homes, like hospitals, require a physician's order for admission. Unlike the decision to admit to a hospital, where the physician usually is operating with some clear clinical protocols and a defined plan for the patient while in the hospital, the nursing-home decision is a murkier one that often puts the doctor in the middle of ambiguous family controversies. The distinction between these two decisions is an important one. A physician hospitalizing a patient normally has decided that the patient's condition requires the technological intensity or physical facilities of the hospital. Further, the general intent is to keep the person in the hospital for a relatively short span of time. In contrast to the hospital stay, the nursing-home stay might be expected to last for several years, and the facility itself is considerably less sophisticated technologically. In fact, most of what occurs in a nursing home could take place in a person's own home with the help of a dedicated family or paid aides and with certain modifications to the physical environment.

In light of the differences between hospitals and nursing homes, as well as the stigma attached to being in a nursing home, I found it unsurprising to learn from a number of doctors that when it comes to a nursing-home decision, they see themselves playing less of a clinical role and more of a psychosocial support role for the resident and the family. What this means for the practitioners is that they usually are cast in the part of the option raiser, permission giver, or facilitator.

As the option raiser, the physician is dealing with a person or family who either has not thought about the nursing home or has simply dismissed it without recognizing the value of that alternative. For example, one practitioner told me of the case of a widower with chronic heart disease who lived alone and received a great deal of assistance from both local social-service agencies and a daughter who lived nearby with her family and also held a full-time job. At some point, it became obvious to both the physician and the daughter that this man needed twenty-four-hour supervision, but it wasn't until the doctor said, "Maybe we should consider a nursing home" that the topic became a legitimate subject for discussion.

In a closely related role, the physician is cast as the person who gives the family permission to do what any objective, disinterested observer would acknowledge has to be done. A frequent problem that the physician encounters when acting as the permission giver is that of handling the assertion, "Going into a nursing home is going to kill my mother." Two common responses are: "You will be amazed at how easily she adjusts to the home" and "It really is in her best interests." Not dealt with here is the often present and unarticulated sense of enormous guilt felt by families who place someone in a nursing home. In fact, few people "die" from moving to a nursing home, most adjust to their new environments, and if the home is the only sensible option, then it needs to be exercised.

A third role the physician may play is that of facilitator. Here although the soon-to-be resident and the family have decided that a nursing home is the best option available, they do not know which of several homes would be best. The doctor is then placed in the position of suggesting several homes and perhaps telling the family what he thinks of each of them. As facilitators, physicians sometimes find themselves in the situation of trying to portray a person in a more attractive light in order to facilitate admission to a desirable home. One physician, who carefully medicated an obstreperous patient with tranquilizers prior to a nursing-home interview, described himself in this case as a coconspirator with the family.

In sum, from a purely clinical perspective, virtually every physician with whom I spoke agreed that there are plenty of patients who receive skilled-nursing care at home, but once the support systems start to fall apart, or the demands become too much for the support systems, then a nursing home becomes the best alternative.

THE BUREAUCRATIC PERSPECTIVE

Before someone goes into a nursing home, at least one and perhaps several bureaucracies may have to be dealt with, including the nursing home's admissions staff and, if the resident is a Medicaid recipient, a representative from the Medicaid bureau. Basically, everyone involved in the admissions process is looking at the same issues: whether a person's needs are such that a nursing home is the right place and what level of care the person needs.

In general, these needs are measured by activity of daily living (ADL) scales, which examine six areas of possible dependency: (1) bathing, (2) dressing, (3) using the toilet, (4) transferring—that is, getting into and out of bed or a chair, (5) bowel and bladder control (continence), and (6) eating. There is also a secondary scale that addresses the needs of the elderly, but usually is not applied to nursing-home needs because it focuses on skills involved in being independent and managing in a community. This scale, called the instrumental activities of daily living (IADL), has a number of components that evaluate the difficulty a person has with the routine tasks of daily living, such as shopping, doing laundry, taking medications, going for a walk, and cleaning up the house.

For the new resident who will pay privately, the process usually is fairly streamlined. In such cases, the agreement for institutionalization and level of care is made between the nursing home and the individual or his/her representative. But in many instances, being ready, willing, and able to pay does not guarantee admission—particularly in a situation where beds are not readily available. Also, in some states, regardless of how the bill will be paid, the state must approve the level of care placement—the rationale being that someday the resident could run out of private funds and the state would have to pick up the bill, so it wants to be sure the placement is correct from the start. Finally, under present federal legislation, all new admissions must be prescreened for mental illness and mental retardation. This program started in 1989 and is under court challenge, but it, too, has the potential for slowing the admissions process. (The actual admissions policy statement of a high-quality nursing home is at the end of this chapter.)

On a private-pay admission, it may be necessary to demonstrate a "need" for care, which is likely to be determined by a member of the nursing home's social-service or admitting staff. In general, these people are looking for a new resident who needs the home's services but will not become an inordinate drain on its resources.

The determination of need for care will be made from data generated from several sources. One source will be a summary medical report provided by the prospective resident's physician. This report will ask for current diagnoses, past medical and surgical history, such other basic medical information as allergies and immunizations, and the recent report of a physician. Frequently the doctor will be asked to provide information about a person's family and/or social history and data about medications and diet.

A second source of information comes from the application

form. These forms (examples of which appear at the end of this chapter) typically request information about the applicant's social and clinical background as well as financial resources. The third and perhaps more significant data source is that generated by the nursing home from an interview with the prospective resident and his or her family. This interview will probe the prospective resident's ability or lack of ability to handle the activities of daily living—most particularly, bathing, toileting, dressing, ambulating, eating, and transferring. Additionally, the interviewers place emphasis on the person's cognitive state, and some institutions even run the prospective resident through an evaluation. Finally, there is a subjective dimension, which does not ask whether the applicant needs the home but rather whether the applicant will "fit into" the home. The answer to that question is equally important, since no home wishes to burden itself with a disruptive resident (or family) for the several years that he or she is likely to be there.

The prospective resident who is a Medicaid recipient and is hospitalized may have a shortcut into the nursing home. If the doctor determines that the patient should be in a nursing home, the hospital's discharge planners and social workers usually will prepare the person for the nursing home and even go so far as to arrange the placement. When the hospital staff goes through this process of determining a person's need for care, it usually is merely countersigned by the Medicaid bureau, which has essentially delegated the determination of need to the hospital staff. For the prospective resident and his or her family, the problem with this is the pressure to accept the home the hospital has selected. Refusing to use that home places them at risk of having no nursing-home bed and potentially continuing in the hospital but being responsible for some portion of the bill.

The last possibility is that a person presently living outside of an institution now needs to be in a nursing home. In such a situation, the Medicaid bureau sends a field worker to the private home to determine the person's eligibility for care. Although there appears to be a scoring system to quantify the data, in practice the scoring system is not used, and it is the judgment of the field worker, normally a nurse, that results in a decision. If the applicant's physician agrees with the field

worker's decision, the placement proceeds. In the case of disagreement, there is an appeals process.

In the most common situation, an individual is already eligible for Medicaid and his or her health condition has dete-
riorated to such a point that family members can no longer be
the caregivers. Medicaid is called, a field worker is dispatched,
and a determination is made within a week or so that the
person is a skilled- or intermediate-care case. Once the level is
determined, the individual is essentially certified and the family can proceed to look for a nursing home. Sometimes a family places the person in the home first and the determination
comes later. Obviously, such an approach runs the risk of a
denial, in which case, the family or the resident may be personally liable for the nursing-home bill.

When the Medicaid staff denies a nursing-home placement
for someone, it usually is because some less expensive
alternative—such as adult foster care, rest-home, or home
health care—is available. In Massachusetts, for example, when
this occurs, the Medicaid branch takes on the responsibility of
helping the recipient find proper alternative services.

CONCLUSION

Despite various attempts to define the concept of need objectively, in the end it still remains an elusive idea and a subjective decision. The American health and social-service system
is at times illogical, such as with the Massachusetts adult
foster-care program that will pay strangers $525 a month (tax
free) to care for the elderly in their home but will not give
either a dime or a tax break to a family that provides the same
care to one of its own. Clearly, a fair percentage of persons in
nursing homes could be cared for outside of those facilities if
there were adequate support systems in terms of family, social, and health agencies. On the other hand, those people
who are in the nursing homes are probably there because no
other alternative was realistically possible.

NURSING HOME   Pg __1__ of __5__
POLICIES AND PROCEDURES
TITLE: __ADMISSIONS__   Date issued _____
DEPT.   __ADMINISTRATION__   Date revised _____

I. PURPOSE:

The purpose of this policy is to establish the requirements for admission to the _____ Nursing Home _____ and to outline the procedures for application and admission.

II. POLICY:

The admission policies of the _____ Nursing Home are based on the belief that the Home furnishes to the communities it serves needed services in the areas of health care, nutritional care, rehabilitative and social programs in a relaxed homelike environment.

Admission to the Home shall be primarily based on a diagnostic study of the physical, social and emotional needs of the applicant. The applicant shall be able to utilize and benefit from the services offered by the Home.

The financial ability of the applicant or the family shall not be utilized as a criteria for admission to the Home. The individual, however, must either meet the criteria for private pay or public assistance.

All information, applications, and related materials and conversations shall be held in the strictest of confidence by the Home and its staff. Care and consideration will be taken with each applicant to assure confidentiality in the processing of the application.

The Home shall not discriminate on admission by race, creed, sex, age, handicap, color, religion, national origin, sources of referral, or source of payment. The Home shall comply with State and Federal antidiscrimination laws. Admission shall be based on applicant need and bed availability, and shall conform to State admission criteria.

III. AGE:

The general minimum age for admission shall be 65 years of age. However, other individuals may be accepted if they have need or benefit from the Home's services. Individuals under 22 years of age may only be admitted with prior approval of the Medical Review Team of the Department of Public Health.

NURSING HOME   Pg __2__ of __5__
POLICIES AND PROCEDURES

TITLE: ___ADMISSIONS___   Date issued _____

DEPT. ___ADMINISTRATION___   Date revised _____

RESIDENCY:

There is no residency requirement. However, priority will be given to applicants, or their families, who reside in _____.

MARITAL STATUS:

Applicants will be accepted from individuals or married couples. If one member of the couple is in need of the services of the Home and meets all requirements, then the requirements (other than financial considerations) may be waived for the other spouse.

HEALTH:

Consideration shall be given to applicants where it is believed the facilities and services of the Home can contribute to the physical and mental well-being of the individual or can effectively meet the applicant's needs. Cases will be accepted compatible with the availability of the appropriate bed and Home staffing.

Excluded from admission shall be those suffering from:

1. A communicable contagious or infectious disease beyond the Home's ability to provide care.
2. Those whose behavior is unmanageable and who may be a detriment to themselves or others.
3. Individuals whose *major* problem is addiction to or dependence on narcotics, alcohol, stimulants, hallucinogenic drugs or other habit-forming drugs.
4. Individuals who, based on an initial evaluation either by the Home, the Department of Public Welfare, Department of Mental Health or Department of Mental Retardation, are inappropriate for nursing home placement.

MEDICAL REQUIREMENTS:

1. Residents recently admitted from the hospital shall have the hospital provide the Home a discharge summary or completed medical evaluation.
2. Applicants will be required to authorize the Home to obtain medical records from attending physicians and/or other health care facilities.

IV. ADMISSION PROCEDURES:

A. Inquiries regarding admission should be addressed to the Social Service Office or Administration.

NURSING HOME   Pg ___3___ of ___5___
POLICIES AND PROCEDURES

TITLE: __ADMISSIONS__   Date issued _____
DEPT.   __ADMINISTRATION__   Date revised _____

B. Applicants and/or other interested parties should be encouraged to visit the Home to review the applicant procedures and to see the facility.

C. During the application process the Social Service staff shall provide a full explanation of the admission procedures, eligibility requirements, services offered and financial policies.

D. The completed application and all the accompanying forms, including medical reports must be returned prior to admission.

E. A representative of the Social Service staff will arrange a visit to meet the proposed resident for the purpose of assessing the applicant's required level of care. A nurse, therapist or other professional staff member may accompany the social worker on the visit.

F. Applicants applying for Medicaid benefits will be required to be seen by a representative of the Case Management section of the Department of Public Welfare for an assessment of the need for skilled or intermediate care services. Determination will also be made for level of care. Application for Medicaid benefits should be made immediately.

G. Applicants not applying for Medicaid benefits may choose not to be evaluated by a representative of the Department of Public Welfare for an assessment as to the need for skilled or intermediate care services. At the time of admission the applicant and/or applicant's representative will sign a waiver which will be kept in the social service record.

H. Upon completion of all application procedures, the applicant will be placed on the Home's waiting list.

I. The exact date of admission will be determined by staff, based on bed availability, applicant need, other extenuating circumstances and/or time on the waiting list.

J. While on the waiting list, Social Services staff will remain in contact with the applicant.

K. On the date of admission the Social Service staff will assist the new resident in his or her transition to the Home. At that time a residency contract will be executed.

NURSING HOME   Pg __4__ of __5__
POLICIES AND PROCEDURES
TITLE: __ADMISSIONS__   Date issued _____
DEPT.   __ADMINISTRATION__   Date revised _____

L. All individuals applying for admission to the nursing home, regardless of payment method, are subject to the preadmission screening requirements of Section 1919 (e) (7) of the Social Security Act as amended by the Omnibus Budget Reconciliation Act of 1987 (OBRA). The purpose is to protect the rights of all residents in nursing homes and to ensure that they receive appropriate care and treatment. The OBRA legislation seeks to ensure that persons with a current primary or secondary diagnosis of a major mental illness as defined in the DSM-IIIR, or who are mentally retarded and/or developmentally disabled are appropriately placed in skilled or intermediate nursing care facilities.

M. Applicants applying for Medicaid benefits, who have a major mental disorder, mental retardation or a developmental disability as defined in OBRA-87, will require a comprehensive assessment prior to admission to determine that placement in the nursing home is appropriate, and if the applicant is in need of active treatment. The comprehensive assessment will be completed by a mental health provider designated by the Department of Mental Health/Department of Mental Retardation.

N. In compliance with OBRA regulations, when the applicant is not applying for Medicaid benefits, prior to admission a waiver (identification screening for nonrecipients waiving LTCC screening) will be completed by designated professional staff of the _____ Nursing Home. The waiver will be kept on the chart.

O. When the applicant (not applying for Medicaid benefits) has a major mental illness and there are no exemptions as stated in Section II of the Waiver, the Department of Mental Health (508-745-2440) will be notified to fulfill OBRA requirements for a comprehensive assessment prior to admission.

P. When the applicant (not applying for Medicaid benefits) is mentally retarded or has a developmental disability and there are no exemptions the Department of Mental Retardation (731-7742, Ext. 237) will be notified to arrange for a comprehensive assessment prior to admission.

NURSING HOME   Pg __5__ of __5__
POLICIES AND PROCEDURES
TITLE: ___ADMISSIONS___   Date issued _____
DEPT. ___ADMINISTRATION___   Date revised _____

Q. When the applicant is not applying for Medicaid benefits, after the Waiver has been completed, if the applicant has a major mental illness, is mentally retarded or developmentally disabled, and has an exemption as stated in Section II of the Waiver, the applicant can be admitted to the _____ Nursing Home without a comprehensive assessment by the Department of Mental Health/Department of Mental Retardation.

SAMPLE SCREENING FORM

Your Department of   Identification Screening for Nonrecipients
Public Welfare   Waiving LTCC Screening

180 Tremont Street
Boston, MA. 02111

This form is to be completed only for those individuals who meet the eligibility criteria for skilled nursing or intermediate care facility services as described in 106 CMR 456.251 through 456.270.

Provider Information Section		Recipient Information Section	
Provider's Name & Address		Recipient's Name & Address	Sex
			☐ M ☐ F
Provider's Telephone No.	Provider No.	Date of Birth	Recipient ID No.
( )			

Section I. Identification

1. Does the individual have a documented diagnosis or treatment history of any of the following major mental disorders?
   - ☐ Schizophrenia   ☐ Paranoia
   - ☐ Major Affective Disorder ☐ Schizoaffective Disorder
   - ☐ Atypical Psychosis   ☐ None of the above

2. Does the individual have a documented diagnosis or treatment history of mental retardation or a related condition?
   ☐ Yes   ☐ No

3. Has the individual ever received inpatient or outpatient psychiatric treatment?
   ☐ Yes   ☐ No

4. Has the individual received services for mental retardation or a related condition from an agency that serves the mentally retarded, the developmentally disabled, or both?
   ☐ Yes   ☐ No

5. Does the individual exhibit any evidence of a major mental illness?
   ☐ Yes   ☐ No

6. Does the individual exhibit any evidence that may indicate mental retardation or a related disorder?
   ☐ Yes   ☐ No

(If you have answered "*No*" to all of the above, skip *Section II* and go on to *Section III.*)

Section II. Exemptions   (Complete only if you answered *"Yes"* to at least one question in *Section I.*)
Does the individual meet any of the following conditions?
☐   Alzheimer's disease or other dementia
☐   Comatose
☐   Ventilator-dependent
☐   Brain-stem level functioning
☐   Chronic obstructive pulmonary disease
☐   Severe Parkinson's disease
☐   Huntington's disease
☐   Amyotrophic lateral sclerosis
☐   Congestive heart failure
☐   Convalescent care not to exceed 120 days following acute hospital stay
☐   Terminal illness certified by physician
☐   None of the above

Section III. Certification
Based on the above findings I certify that (check one):
☐   There is no indication of mental illness/mental retardation.
☐   Mental illness/mental retardation is indicated, but individual meets one of the exemptions in Section II.
☐   Mental illness/mental retardation is indicated and referral has been made to the appropriate agency for assessment.

Signature _____   Date _____

Title _____

43

ALTERNATIVES TO NURSING HOMES

One question that I have asked hundreds, perhaps thousands, of people is whether they wish to spend the last years of their lives in a nursing home. The clear and unequivocal answer is almost always no. With all the talk and anxiety about nursing homes, one fact is often lost: Most elderly people do not live in them. Indeed, even those with serious physical problems, or significant cognitive functional impairments such as Alzheimer's disease, can live outside of nursing homes if high-quality alternative programs are accessible and available. This chapter describes and analyzes a number of these programs and suggests ways in which people can tap into community resources so prolonged nursing-home residency is either delayed or avoided.

The chapter begins with a description of two interesting alternatives to nursing-home institutionalization—the "On Lok" approach and New York's "Nursing Home Without Walls" program. The subsequent sections focus on the better-known and widely available home-health-care, adult-day-health-care, and hospice programs. Finally, this chapter concludes with some comments on independent and assisted living alternatives.

THE "ON LOK" APPROACH

An elderly person lucky enough to live in San Francisco's Chinatown, or about ten other locations throughout the country, may be able to take advantage of a unique response to the problems of aging by joining the On Lok program. *On Lok* is a Chinese word that means "abode of peace and happiness," epitomizing the philosophy of the organization.

Since the early 1970s, the On Lok program has organized and operated a high-quality, 300-bed nursing home without the physical facility of resident rooms. Its director, Marie-Louise Ansak, a nationally recognized leader in gerontology, describes the program she developed as "a nursing home on wheels." What this means in practice is that each morning as many as eighty-five On Lok staff members go out to the homes of the frail elderly, assist them in getting out of bed, using the toilet, and dressing for the trip to the On Lok Adult Day Health Center. Once at the center, the program participant eats, perhaps takes a bath, and becomes involved in various therapeutic services and activities. At the end of the day, the individual is driven home with an evening meal in hand. To complete the cycle, if necessary, a staff member will stop by the participant's home to provide assistance in toileting and in getting into bed.

With a total staff of approximately 300, On Lok provides such services as primary medical care, skilled nursing, physical and occupational therapy, social worker assistance and counseling, and nutritional assistance, as well as a wide range of home-care and personal-care services. All of this is done without the physical facility of a nursing home, although the organization does operate On Lok House, a small apartment block in San Francisco that accommodates fifty-four low-income frail elderly in efficiency units. Approximately 64 percent of the On Lok participants live alone, while 30 percent live with a spouse or relative. All of them are frail elderly who have been certified by California's Department of Health Services as being eligible for nursing-home care.

Overall, the cost of On Lok is slightly below that of a full-time nursing-home placement, and its success is perhaps indicated by the fact that the federal government has granted the organization and a few similar ones an "On Lok waiver" so that they can receive Medicare and Medicaid funds as if they were inpatient facilities. The beneficial aspect of this program is clear: The participants have the opportunity to live out their lives in familiar surroundings without compromising the quality of their health care.

In recognition of their dramatic success as well as their health-care leadership, On Lok and Marie-Louise Ansak have received national awards and considerable media attention. For those with access to this program, it is well worth investigating as an option to the traditional nursing home.

"NURSING HOME WITHOUT WALLS"

New Yorkers and residents of the several other states experimenting with the Nursing Home Without Walls program may be eligible for an option that is similar in concept to On Lok. Approximately 8,000 New York residents, most of whom are Medicaid recipients, participate in this program, which was the inspiration of New York State Senator Tarky Lombardi. As with On Lok, its aim is to keep at home people who are prime candidates for admission to nursing homes.

Basically, as with the On Lok approach, services are provided in therapy centers and at home. The difference appears to be that the more extensive New York system tends to function by contracting with a wide variety of not-for-profit, governmental, and for-profit providers, including home-care agencies, hospitals, nursing homes, and other social-service organizations. Thus, the centralized organization and delivery of the On Lok program is not present. At the moment, the program is operating in more than fifty of New York's sixty-two counties and appears to have the capacity to accept new participants in some locations.

The typical patient is a female, over the age of seventy-five, with health-care needs that, but for the program, would normally be provided in a skilled-nursing facility. While the majority of program participants live with family members, it is estimated that 46 percent are living alone. Finally, what is perhaps most interesting from a policy perspective is that this program appears to be treating patients with an array of problems similar to those that would be found in a typical nursing home, including Alzheimer's disease—all at less cost than a comparable nursing-home stay.

HOME HEALTH CARE

Medicare coverage for home health care is not for custodial or maintenance care but rather for therapeutic services. In practice, this means that Medicare will pay for home-health-care services under very strict guidelines when those services are required by someone who is essentially confined to the home and has a medical necessity for skilled-nursing services or physical, occupational, or speech therapy on a regular basis. Under the most recent legislation, a prior hospitalization is not necessary to be eligible for Medicare-covered home care.

In general, this means that people are covered for home care during a short recovery period following hospitalization, when they might need some follow-up restorative therapy for conditions such as hip fractures or acute episodes of a congestive heart condition. If Medicare certifies someone as eligible for home care, the care must be delivered through a home-health-care agency approved and certified by Medicare.

Assuming a patient is receiving one of the therapeutic services, he or she may also be able to receive the part-time services of a home-health aide, occupational therapist, and social-service worker.

If Medicare does not cover the visits, a family can organize its own home-health-care program, although this can be more expensive than nursing-home costs. For example, a typical certified home-care agency may charge upwards of $65 for a visit by a licensed nurse or therapist. Such visits typically last twenty to thirty minutes, although some may be longer and others very short. Aides or companions who have completed two-week training programs may cost in the neighborhood of $15 per hour. People who can help out with shopping, cooking, and other household activities may cost in excess of $12 an hour through these agencies. Families attempting to put together their own programs may also find assistance through friends or perhaps advertisements in local newspapers.

Another aspect of the home-health-care option has to do with medical supplies and equipment, which can, if medically necessary and approved by Medicare, be paid for under Part B of Medicare. (See chapter 4 for an in-depth explanation of the Medicare and Medicaid systems.) The system basically works as follows: The patient's physician files a form attesting to the medical necessity of the equipment, such as a wheelchair or a hospital bed. If the request is approved by Medicare, the government rents the equipment for the patient. There must be a recertification every twelve months, and if approved, the equipment stays in the person's home until it no longer is needed. Inexpensive equipment—which currently is defined as anything costing less than $150—is purchased by the government and given to the patient for his or her use and subsequent disposal. Most reusable supplies are not covered unless they have a particular therapeutic necessity (such as ostomy bags).

The major limitation to approval for equipment is whether it is therapeutically necessary, in which case it is covered; or whether it is for the ease of the caregiver, in which case it is not covered. For example, if the patient is frail and it is simply easier for the caregiver to have the patient use a commode than to walk the patient to the toilet, the commode would not be covered.

The cost of owning or renting medical equipment is such that many families may choose, even with Medicare payment, to set up their own mini–nursing facility at home. Toilets can be modified with grab bars and other devices to raise their heights; showers and tubs can be fitted with grab bars; ramps can be built; cabinetry can be lowered; doorways can be widened; and hospital beds can be utilized. Obviously, while equipment does not support the patient's emotional needs, the availability of durable medical equipment does present an opportunity for some families to keep a relative out of a nursing home.

If a family exercises the option to keep someone at home, various community agencies—in particular, the local area Agency on Aging—often can provide support in the form of meals-on-wheels programs, visitors, transportation, and chore services.

ADULT DAY-CARE PROGRAMS

For many families, nursing homes can be either avoided or postponed thanks to the availability of day-care programs for the elderly. These programs—which go by a variety of names, including geriatric day centers, adult health-care centers, and adult day care—provide a wide range of clinical, nutritional, recreational, and social support services.

Clinical services may include therapies such as physical, occupational, or speech; visits to a primary-care nurse or even a physician; and counseling with a social worker. Nutritional services usually include a well-balanced midday meal, snacks, sometimes meals to take home, and, if appropriate, nutritional counseling. The recreational and social support activities might include gardening therapy, an art program, exercise activities, and a crafts program. Frequently an adult day-care program also will organize transportation for participants.

These types of comprehensive centers are owned and operated by nursing homes, church and community groups, and governmental agencies. Funding usually is provided by a mix of Medicaid and private payments. For many families, a day-care center is the solution to the problem of keeping an elderly family member at home. It allows other family members the time to pursue their normal activities while ensuring that the elderly person has a safe and stimulating environment for part of a day—all at a cost dramatically below that of a nursing home.

The day-care centers that I visited, all of which were attached to nursing homes, were uniformly bright and cheerful places. Three features always struck me on these visits: First, the abundance of plants seemed to testify that there was universal agreement about the value of garden therapy. Second, I was invariably impressed by the quality of the day-care centers' physical facilities, which usually included dayrooms and numerous sitting places with card tables, sofas, and chairs. Finally, every place I visited had small nutrition/snack kitchens for supplementing the meals that came from the central kitchen; several centers had small rooms with cots for midday naps. Typically, the program participants were sitting in small groups at tables working on arts-and-crafts projects. Their schedules often approximated those of nursing homes and included the usual music activities, exercise classes, discussion groups, and the occasional passive activity, such as a film. Some centers operated their own vans, which picked up and delivered participants; others relied on area Agency on Aging transportation or family members.

SENIOR CENTERS

The adult day-care centers, which number approximately 1,500 and assist approximately 50,000 people, should not be confused with senior centers. Senior-center programs are not alternatives to nursing homes; rather, they are social-activity and educational programs for people over a specific age—which varies by community but usually is in the sixty-plus category.

The health care provided at such centers involves periodic screening programs for glaucoma, high blood pressure, and cholesterol levels. Some programs run transportation systems to help people get around town in order to do grocery shopping or visit local physicians or dentists. Additionally, all centers organize activity programs that include fitness classes, dancing, music, arts and crafts, educational lectures, and, if a pool is available, "senior swims." Some communities have even organized senior travel clubs that make day and weekend excursions. Finally, lunch is often available at these centers through a meals-on-wheels program. Overall, these programs are exceedingly valuable in breaking down any social isolation that an elderly person may face. Unfortunately, they do not offer the range of clinical services that would allow them to be considered as alternatives to nursing homes.

HOSPICES

For some, nursing-home care is considered because of a terminal illness. But there is another alternative that may be much more attractive for those in such a situation: the hospice. The modern hospice movement started in 1968 with the activities of Dr. Cecily Saunders at St. Christopher's Hospice in London. Over the years, her ideas have spread across the Atlantic, landing first in New Haven, Connecticut, in 1974. Today, hospices can be found in more than a thousand communities throughout the country.

The constituency for hospices is dying patients and their families. In the service of a "good death," the hospice staff utilizes the high technology of drug therapy to offer patients a minimum of pain, along with constant personal and emotional attention. The literature is full of stories of staff members hugging and kissing the dying and their families, praying with them, respecting their privacy, and, of course, sharing their grief.

Hospices themselves come in a variety of organizational configurations. For example, some are attached to nursing homes or hospitals, others are freestanding institutions, while still others are basically home-care organizations delivering services to the patient at the domicile. Hospice care, up to a lifetime limit of 210 days, is now covered under Medicare Part A, which will pay for the skilled-nursing care, various therapies, and a percentage of the prescription drug bills.

ALTERNATIVE LIVING ARRANGEMENTS

Many of today's best nursing homes started out decades ago as what is now called "assisted living facilities." In simple language, this meant they provided minimal services to the elderly. Such services might include meal preparation and minimal assistance with some of the activities of daily living, such as dressing and bathing.

Today the elderly have a broad choice of living alternatives. At one end of the spectrum are the upscale retirement villages, such as USAA Towers in San Antonio, Presbyterian Village in Dallas, and Duncaster in Bloomfield, Connecticut. These and many others like them appeal to an affluent population that is looking for a retirement community with large, well-constructed apartments or townhouses and a range of hotel-type services, such as dining rooms, housekeeping assistance, concierges, game rooms, and hobby areas. These same people, many of whom are in their seventies, also purchase some degree of health-care security by moving into these communities, which have such built-in amenities as security systems, medical-alert communication systems, wellness clinics, and nursing-home "connections."

The nature of this nursing home "connection" varies by facility and program. At one end of the spectrum is the "Type A" continuing-care retirement community. Duncaster, which is located in the rolling hills of northern Connecticut, is an excellent example of this type of operation. Duncaster requires a nonrefundable entrance fee of approximately $140,000 for a two-bedroom apartment, plus a monthly maintenance fee of approximately $3,000 for two people. The entrance and maintenance fees cover limited housekeeping, one meal per day, a broad range of activities, and a guarantee of nursing-home care for life at no additional charge.

Another option is the "Type B" communities that, while having both retirement living and a nursing home on the same campus, provide only a limited amount of nursing-home care as part of the package. For example, at Presbyterian Village and USAA Towers, residents are entitled to fourteen days of nursing care per year at the community's nursing facilities (these days are not cumulative). After that, they must pay for the remainder of the required nursing-home stay at full rates. As should be expected, the prices of these options vary considerably. For example, USAA Towers, which is organized as a cooperative apartment complex, costs a minimum of $147,000 for a two-bedroom, two-bath apartment, plus a monthly maintenance fee of $955 for two people. The maintenance fee covers weekly housekeeping, one meal daily per person, such amenities as a health club and swimming pool, plus fourteen days of nursing-home care per year. The initial cost of the apartment is recoverable through a buy-back plan or an open-market sale.

A few hundred miles away, Presbyterian Village operates with a different approach. For an initial payment of approximately $85,000 and a monthly maintenance fee of $1,070, two persons can live in a two-bedroom townhouse. The $85,000 is defined as a prepaid lease on the townhouse and is not refundable (although if a person leaves within the first two years, there is a provision for a prorated refund). As with USAA Towers, the monthly fee covers the usual interior and exterior maintenance of the facility, a range of amenities, plus one meal per day. Also like USAA Towers, a nursing home is attached to the community and residents are entitled to fourteen days of free care per year, the remainder to be paid on a fee-for-service basis.

For those interested in examining the continuing-care retirement community option, the February 1990 *Consumer Reports* should be required reading. In this issue, the staff presents an excellent overview and analysis of these communities along with useful examples. Another valuable source of information about continuing-care retirement communities is the Continuing Care Accreditation Commission, 1129 Twentieth Street, N.W., Suite 400, Washington, DC 20036; telephone (202) 296-5960. At the same address and phone number, you will also find the American Association of Homes for the Aging, which is the primary source of information about the not-for-profit nursing-home community.

There are numerous variations on these themes for people of all economic levels. For example, through a U.S. Department of Housing and Urban Development program, many nursing homes were able to build subsidized housing for the elderly. But be aware that even though many of these housing facilities may be on the grounds of a nursing home, there may be no guarantee of admission to that home, nor is there any commitment to fund the nursing-home stay. What this means in practice is that the proximity of the nursing home may provide only a degree of psychological comfort plus some supportive services such as screening clinics, nutritional counseling, and perhaps meals and entertainment. Paying for the nursing-home care will be a separate issue that will still require navigating the Medicare, Medicaid, or private-payment labyrinth.

If a person is too frail or dependent for independent living but does not require the assistance of a nursing home, then what may be needed is a congregate-care facility. The places of this type that I visited were all quite similar. Typically, they provided private living quarters that had either one or two rooms and a private bathroom. Each section of the facility had a small kitchenette for minor cooking activities and meals were provided in a central dining commons. Staff members were available round the clock to provide what I would classify as minimal but important assistance (such as buttoning shirts or dresses). In general, these congregate-care options offered full housekeeping and laundry services and a variety of activities and excursions.

An option that has gained increased attention because of its problems is the board-and-care facility. These rest homes or personal-care beds typically provide housing, meals, and minimal supervision for the elderly. In a February 1989 report about these facilities, the U.S. General Accounting Office (GAO) estimated that there were 41,000 licensed homes with 563,000 beds and an unknown number of unlicensed beds. The GAO report, as well as other research, suggests that serious problems frequently exist with these homes in terms of supervision of residents, resident abuse, medication oversight, and improper hygiene and nutrition.

Finally, in what may be considered either a decentralized congregate-care program or perhaps a return to the extended family, some communities and states are experimenting with programs under which the elderly are placed with foster families. In Massachusetts, more than 200 elderly persons are in such a program, which involves moving in with a foster family that provides housing, meals, and some minimal assistance—reminding the person to take medications, for example. In return for the psychosocial assistance to an elderly person, foster families in Massachusetts receive a monthly stipend of $525—considerably less cost for the state than a nursing-home placement.

Overall, it appears that there are a number of options other than nursing homes if an elderly person is basically healthy and able to function more or less independently. However, once the independent functioning is gone, then one of the nursing-home options is likely to be exercised unless family members are able to set up and adequately staff their own home or the home of the elderly family member. In response to this need, the Canadians and Australians have encouraged the development of "granny flats," which essentially are specially designed mobile homes temporarily attached to one's home to allow a family to care for an elderly member but also maintain space and privacy. When the best alternative is indeed the nursing home, the choice of a nursing home becomes crucial. The next chapters of this book are designed to assist elderly people and their families in dealing with the issues of paying for care, assessing the quality of care, and making the best possible choice.

FOUR

PAYING FOR NURSING-HOME CARE

The issue is a simple one: Who is going to pay the $30,000 per year nursing home bill? Despite myriad misconceptions, Medicare usually won't; Medicaid might if the resident is poor enough; and, in the end, the family may be left holding the bag. This chapter provides an overview of the options for financing nursing-home care and identifies what steps a family should take to clarify eligibility for public payment for care. The following chapter looks at the special issues relating to financing nursing-home care including admissions fees, doctor bills, private-duty nurses and helpers, and additional hidden costs such as telephone and laundry expenses.

MEDICARE

Elderly people and their families generally believe Medicare will pay most nursing-home bills. This misconception was probably reinforced with the hoopla surrounding President Ronald Reagan's signing of the Catastrophic Coverage Act of 1988. Fueling this confusion were the statements of such politicians as the Democratic senator from Texas and sponsor of the bill, Lloyd Bentsen, who said, "What we're doing is saying to the elderly that the nightmare that you feared so much if you have a catastrophic illness you're going to have your life savings wiped out . . . that's going to be taken care of." Senator Bentsen was not alone in sending out mixed messages about this amendment to the Medicare legislation. Senator John Chafee, Republican from Rhode Island, stated, "This vote will give the elderly long-overdue peace of mind." And Senator Barbara Mikulski, Democrat from Maryland, added that the bill would prevent the elderly from going into financial ruin and that the bill was "greatly needed to shore up the safety net for seniors."

Despite these statements from politicians, this bill probably should have been called the Election Year Acute Care Catastrophic Coverage Act. Such a label would have been more accurate since the primary focus of the 1988 bill was on insuring the elderly against being wiped out by a long hospital stay. The unfortunate reality is that over the years Medicare has provided minimal nursing-home coverage; indeed, it has covered only about 2 percent of the bills for nursing-home care.

Medicare is structured as a two-part health insurance system for people over sixty-five and those who have certain disabilities or chronic diseases, such as kidney failure. The first part of the system, called "Part A," is essentially a hospital insurance program. Like any other hospital insurance program, it collects premiums, sets limits on what it will pay, has deductibles, and has all kinds of rules. For example, Medicare covers semiprivate accommodations, meals (including special diets), laboratory and X-ray testing, operating room charges, and drug costs while in the hospital. Examples of costs that would not be covered would be telephone charges and private-duty nurses a patient or family orders for convenience or for peace of mind.

The confusion about the Medicare and nursing-home coverage exists because the government, as a prudent buyer of health services, decided that in some instances it would be cheaper to pay for the equivalent of hospital services in a less expensive facility—that is, in a skilled-nursing home. So for many years Medicare provided up to 100 days in a skilled-nursing facility if certain requirements were met. The two prime requirements were: (1) The Medicare beneficiary went to the nursing home subsequent to a recent hospital stay for the same condition the home was going to treat; and, (2) the services to be provided were, as discussed in chapter 1, of a skilled nature. These requirements also meant that Medicare would not pay for maintenance and custodial care, which is what most of nursing-home care is all about. Another and perhaps simpler way of looking at this is that under the old Medicare rules the skilled-nursing facility was functioning as an extension of the hospital, and the Medicare program would pay for the totality of what could theoretically be a hospital stay, whether care was given in the hospital or in the nursing home.

The provisions of the 1988 Catastrophic Coverage Act fundamentally deepened the coverage but did not broaden it. Thus, the old provisions that limited care to 100 days was changed to cover 150 days in skilled-nursing facilities. A technically confusing area called "spell of illness" was eliminated. And, perhaps of greatest importance, the requirement for a prior hospitalization before admittance into a skilled-nursing facility was eliminated. Thus, after the 1988 Act was implemented, someone who qualified for Part A Medicare benefits for a skilled-nursing home would not have to first be admitted to a hospital before being allowed into a rehabilitation program in a nursing home and be covered by Medicare.

Unfortunately, on the day before Thanksgiving 1989, Congress repealed the Catastrophic Coverage Act of 1988. This repeal was in response to an outcry from Medicare beneficiaries who felt that they were being overburdened by the extra premiums associated with the 1988 Act. What this repeal means is that to qualify for Medicare coverage in a skilled-nursing facility a person must have a three-day prior hospitalization before transfer to a nursing home and the transfer must, usually, occur within thirty days of that hospitalization. Coverage for a resident of a skilled-nursing facility is limited to 100 days per benefit period; (there is normally a sixty-day break between benefit periods); and for the first twenty days Medicare pays 100 percent of approved charges and for the next eighty days there is a $74.00 per day deductible.

None of this, however, deals with the actual process of qualifying for nursing-home benefits under Medicare. In fact, the process remained essentially unaltered. As before, it had to start with a physician ordering covered services that might be broadly classified as either rehabilitative physical therapy or extended skilled-nursing care such as for patients receiving intravenous fluids or gastrostomy feedings. In both instances the doctor's orders become the vehicle for the hospital discharge and placement in a nursing home. In addition, for the services to be paid for by Medicare they must be provided to a Medicare beneficiary in a Medicare-certified Level I facility. To qualify for payment for the rehabilitative services, the patient would have to be receiving daily physical therapy treatment and have the potential to be discharged to home. While many different conditions and services qualify for skilled-nursing care, a key criterion is: "The daily skilled services must be such that, as a practical matter, they can only be provided in a SNF, on an inpatient basis."

In an attempt to clarify what is meant by "practical matter," the federal regulations indicated that those who approve the Medicare claims should consider whether the patient's condition really warrants a skilled-nursing facility and whether options exist other than a skilled-nursing facility that would be more economical and feasible. Further, there was the ominous phrase in the regulation that ". . . in making that determination, the availability of Medicare payment for those services may not be a factor." The example the regulations provided to illustrate this point was that of a beneficiary who can receive daily physical therapy services from a physical therapist in private practice. On the other hand, the regulations did indicate that the difficulty of transporting a person daily to therapy may be enough to make Medicare-financed skilled-nursing facility alternative the best choice.

If all of this sounds confusing, that's because it is. Some nursing-home social workers and utilization review coordinators I talked to said they had absolutely no problem with the stipulation that post-hospital residents who were coming in for physical therapy have the potential to be discharged to home. The world is grayer when one talks of the person who merely needs twenty-four-hour supervision as a post–heart attack case. One senior official in the Medicare program acknowledged that there is considerable variability throughout the country in how the program is applied. This comes about because the decision-making on Medicare status is not done centrally in Washington, but rather on a totally decentralized basis. In fact, Medicare contracts with insurance companies to act as fiscal intermediaries between the Medicare beneficiaries and the government. For example, it is quite possible for a claim to be turned down in one state and approved in another. Indeed, in this senior official's own family an elderly relative spent several weeks in a New Jersey nursing home before Medicare disallowed his skilled-nursing facility claim—a claim that the official is certain would have been approved in his home state of Maryland.

Further confounding the Medicare payment issue is the program's second component, Part B, which is voluntary and requires a supplemental payment. Part B covers a portion of the doctor bills, diagnostic testing such as lab work and X-rays, and in some instances physical, occupational, or speech therapies. The way Part B operates, the patient must pay the premium for enrollment, cover an annual deductible that changes from year to year, and then pay 20 percent of the charges for whatever the service. The Part B program also limits the number of routine visits for which it will pay, although there is no limit for visits related to a specific illness or injury. But Part B, like Part A, does not pay the routine costs of care in a nursing home—so it too does not pay the $30,000 bill.

In sum, Medicare remains the primary payer of hospital bills for the elderly but, unfortunately, Medicare cannot be looked to as a source of insurance for custodial nursing-home care.

On the other hand, Medicaid, the health program for the impoverished or medically needy, will pick up the bill for a patient who qualifies. The next section examines the role of Medicaid in paying for nursing-home care.

MEDICAID

In its October 3, 1988, issue, *People* magazine featured the story of Celia Goldie, a ninety-year-old woman who had moved from her condo on Chicago's North Shore to a nursing home in suburban Skokie. The article pointed out that prior to moving into the nursing home, Mrs. Goldie—a widow with a married and apparently devoted son—had been living on financial thin ice. Her $25,000 in savings had been depleted by expenses for aides and housekeepers, who were needed after she had a heart attack and stroke three years earlier, and her $597 monthly Social Security income did not cover her $700 mortgage and maintenance payments, nor her grocery bills and the salary of her $160-per-week companion. The move to the nursing home meant an end to her crisis and the subsidy provided by her son, because once she was eligible for Medicaid, it would pay for most of her nursing-home costs.

Mrs. Goldie's story is not significantly different from those of hundreds of thousands of others who live middle-class lives but find themselves unable to afford the ever-escalating costs of nursing-home care. Fortunately, the solution is the Medicaid program.

Medicaid is not to be confused with Medicare. As explained in the previous section, Medicare is a federal hospital- and medical-insurance program tied to the Social Security system. Medicaid is a joint state and federal program that provides funding for health services for the needy. The framework for Medicaid comes from a set of federal regulations that were described by Supreme Court Justice Lewis Powell as Byzantine. Another federal judge described the statute as being "unintelligible to the uninitiated." While the federal government provides the framework, it is up to the states to make the decisions about the provision of services and eligibility. The result of all of this "flexibility" is, as already noted regarding the Medicare program, that there also is considerable variability among the states.

At the level of nursing-home owners and managers, the variability comes most importantly in terms of how much the state Medicaid program will reimburse the home for a day of care for a Medicaid recipient. Since federal law prohibits the family or the resident from supplementing the Medicaid payment, this reimbursement becomes the home's primary income for the Medicaid beneficiary, and it must cover the expenses of salaries, supplies, and services. As an example of the state-to-state variability, consider the reimbursements paid to comparable homes that I visited in Dallas, Texas; Kansas City, Missouri; and Fairfield, Connecticut. In Dallas, the reimbursement was $34.60 per day; in Kansas City, $51.60; and in Fairfield, $93.84.

From the perspective of the long-term resident or the potential resident of a nursing home, the threshold question is whether they are eligible for Medicaid. Eligibility will be determined by a local welfare office after gathering information from an applicant about assets and income. In terms of assets, the Medicaid system generally asks about the prospective resident's real and personal property, and if it exceeds the specified maximum, the person must "spend down" to the limit before being eligible. In other words, applicants must deplete their own resources before the government will pay. In terms of income, the income must be used first to offset the nursing-home bill before the Medicaid program will pay. To clarify the issue of eligibility, below are several typical examples, using the 1988 regulations in effect in Massachusetts:

CASE 1

Mrs. W. is a seventy-seven-year-old widow with no children whose only income is $437 per month from Social Security. She lives in a rental apartment with furniture that has a market value of $500. Her jewelry and other personal possessions are worth $2,000. She has no other assets.

Mrs. W. will be eligible because she simply is poor enough. If she chooses to sell off her furniture and other personal possessions and deposit the money in a bank account, she will have a larger than is allowable for Medicaid; she will have to spend down her $2,500 account to the $2,000 limit before she can become eligible again. From her $437 monthly income, Mrs. W. will be allowed to keep $70 per month in a personal account. But if Mrs. W. does sell off her possessions and realize the $2,500, she can shelter the extra $500 by prepaying her funeral expenses and placing up to $2,500 in a funeral-expense account.

CASE 2

Mr. X. is an eighty-three-year-old widower with two adult children; each month he receives a Social Security check of $611 and a private pension check of $150. He has $15,000 in the bank and a house valued at $175,000. In order to qualify for Medicaid, he first has to spend down the $15,000 to reach $2,000. He does this by paying his own nursing-home bill. But, as in the case of Mrs. W., he is allowed to have up to $2,000 in a bank account plus a burial-expense account of up to $2,500. This latter account is merely a bank account that can be held jointly with a child and is earmarked for burial expenses. Mr. X. can also prepay all his funeral expenses, including costs for a gravesite and marker—and there is no limit on this. For our example, we can assume he has paid $7,500 for the funeral, gravesite, monument, and perpetual care at the cemetery. So, from his $15,000, there is now only $3,000, which he gives to his children. Medicaid can now recover that $3,000 that was spent in anticipation of going into the nursing home and have it applied to the nursing-home bill. As far as Mr. X.'s house is concerned, several options exist. One is to sell the house and apply the money toward Mr. X.'s nursing-home bill. If this occurs, Mr. X. probably will spend his years in the nursing home as a private-pay resident. A second option, which was available until 1989, is to transfer the house to a child for no money so that the house is no longer Mr. X.'s asset. A third possibility is to do nothing, and when Mr. X. dies and the house passes into his estate, the state can recover from the estate whatever funds it expended on Mr. X.'s behalf. Finally, it turns out that Mr. X.'s two children are multimillionaires who also live and work in Massachusetts. Will the state attempt to have the children pay the nursing-home bill for their father? In Massachusetts the answer is no. However, there is increasing interest in some states to make children financially more responsible for their parents who are in nursing homes.

One twist on Mr. X.'s story might be that twenty-six months before going into the nursing home and applying for Medicaid, he gave a million dollars to his children. If the transfer occurred two years prior to his entering a nursing home, the state will not count that amount in determining Medicaid eligibility. But if the transfer of funds occurred within two years, Medicaid normally will count the million dollars in making its eligibility determination.

CASE 3

Mr. and Mrs. Z. have stocks and bonds worth $25,000, a house with a market value of $150,000, and different monthly pension incomes. Mr. Z. gets $606 from Social Security while Mrs. Z. receives $213 from Social Security as well as $1,800 from her private pension plan. Mr. Z. is admitted to a nursing home and, after the second month, applies for Medicaid. In this case, Medicaid will first take the stocks and bonds and, unless they are held in one name, split the value between the spouses. Thus, Mr. Z. is now assumed to have $12,500 in liquid assets. With this, Mr. Z. can go ahead with funeral plans and their separate burial-expense accounts. Assuming that when all of that is taken care of, Mr. Z. has assets worth $5,000, he must then spend down to the $2,000 level before Medicaid will kick in with its contribution for the nursing-home care. As in the instance of Mrs. W., Mr. Z. will have to turn over his Social Security check, which will essentially be the first dollars to be paid to the nursing home, but he will be able to keep $70 per month for his personal account. Mrs. Z. gets to keep half the stocks and bonds, the house, and the car (assuming there is one), plus her pension checks.

These three cases are fairly simple examples of how (in 1988) one state was likely to deal with establishing Medicaid eligibility for a nursing-home resident. What should be evident from all of that is the following: (1) The laws governing eligibility are confusing and complex; (2) each state determines eligibility differently; and (3) the determination for eligibility is made by local Medicaid staff, so it is important to understand a locality's rules. A cautionary note: Regulations change constantly, so it is essential to do additional investigation on the local level. For example, in order to forestall spousal impoverishment, new government Medicaid eligibility rules are emerging that allow noninstitutionalized spouses to keep up to $60,000 in assets, at least $815 per month of combined family income (although some states such as Massachusetts and Maryland allow as much as $1,500 per month in income), a house and a car. Also the transfer of assets requirements have now been lengthened to a thirty-month look-back or cutoff period.

For an unfortunate number of people, a lifetime of scrimping and saving for the "golden years" winds up being spent in six months or a year in a nursing home. Some families wishing to minimize the risk of losing a lifetime's worth of savings to a long-term-care facility have turned to the option of long-term-care insurance. In the final section of this chapter, I shall explore the ins and outs of this third financing option.

LONG-TERM-CARE INSURANCE

Half of the people in nursing homes are "private pays"—that is, they or members of their families wind up footing the bill. To deal with this enormous financial burden, more than seventy insurance companies have begun to offer long-term-care insurance. Unfortunately, however, this insurance product does not solve many problems—indeed, for the most part, it confuses matters.

To understand the problem with long-term-care insurance, it helps to recognize first that insurance companies are not in business to provide charity; they are financial institutions interested in profits: Profits are generated by collecting premiums and investing those premiums; profits are reduced when insured events occur. To avoid too many high-priced payoffs, they must charge high enough premiums, insure large enough populations, and set payoff conditions. Basically, the insurance company is betting *against* certain events happening and the insured is betting that these events *will* occur. In the case of long-term-care insurance, the "event" that the company must be concerned about is the extremely expensive one of a $30,000 annual nursing-home bill. The insured pays premiums on the off chance of collecting if he or she needs nursing-home care, but the insurance company minimizes its financial exposure in a variety of ways. First, it may set limits on whom it will insure. These limits may be a function of a person's age or health status. It would be bad business, for example, for a company to collect premiums for only two or three months from someone on the verge of entering a nursing home. A second way insurance companies limit financial exposure is by setting premiums at a level that corresponds with age. *Consumer Reports* noted in 1988 that one company, Great Republic, charged a seventy-five-year-old $3,143 per year for a policy that a fifty-five-year-old could buy for $611 per year.

Financial exposure is further limited by companies offering policies that only pay specified benefits, such as $50 or $100 per day for a limited number of days, and that do not begin paying until the beneficiary has been in the nursing home for a certain number of days. And some insurance policies require, as the old Medicare rules did, a related hospitalization prior to the nursing-home stay; or, in some cases, only a certain level of care will be covered. Finally, many of these policies have in them a wide range of exclusions, such as for preexisting conditions, Alzheimer's disease, or any type of dementia.

The conclusion, then, is simple: It is almost impossible for anyone faced with going into a nursing home in the immediate future to obtain insurance that will provide more than token coverage. For long-range planners who are looking for insurance to cover their future needs in their fifties or sixties or perhaps early seventies, the only advice I can give now is to be a very prudent shopper.

Regrettably, because the United States does not have an insurance system that provides for the comprehensive needs of the elderly, the nursing-home bills fall on the shoulders of the residents or their families who, in more than 50 percent of the cases, pay them with private funds. Unfortunately, these bills may neither start nor stop with the $100-per-day charges for room and board. In the next chapter, I shall examine the hidden costs of nursing-home care.

FIVE

THE HIDDEN COSTS OF NURSING HOMES

Nursing homes can nickel and dime people to distraction if they are not prepared for the additional costs that appear all too frequently. Although most of these costs are petty, they can amount to hundreds, thousands, and in some cases tens of thousands of dollars a year. Since this book is attempting to separate reality from myth, the first section of this chapter focuses on the troublesome issue of admissions fees, while subsequent sections consider the other expenses residents and their families should anticipate in connection with a nursing home.

ADMISSIONS FEES

The critical question here is whether a nursing home can require payment of a nonrefundable fee prior to accepting a new resident. The answer is complicated.

If a person is entitled to receive services under the Medicaid or Medicare program, the Nursing Home Reform Act, which was passed by Congress and signed by President Reagan on December 22, 1988, makes it perfectly clear that admissions fees are illegal:

> . . . a nursing facility must—in the case of an individual who is entitled to medical assistance for nursing facility services— not charge, solicit, accept, or receive, in addition to any amount otherwise required to be paid under the State plan under this title, any gift, money, donation, or other consider-

ation as a precondition of admitting (or expediting the admission of) the individual to the facility or as a requirement for the individual's continued stay in the facility.

But what about admissions fees for private-pay residents? For example, could a nursing home that took both private-pay residents and Medicaid beneficiaries require that private-pay applicants donate money to a building fund before they will be admitted? Alternatively, could a donation to the home expedite the admissions process—for example, could it cause someone to jump the waiting list?

The answer to all of these questions is—it depends. There is significant variation from state to state. For example, Connecticut has a tough antidiscrimination law requiring all nursing homes that accept Medicaid recipients to keep a chronological list of applicants and admit them on a first-come, first-served basis, regardless of the source of payment. The Connecticut statute states:

> Each nursing home shall (A) provide a receipt to each applicant for admission to its facility who requests placement on a waiting list stating the date and time of such request and (B) maintain a dated list of such applications which shall be available at all times to any applicant, his bona fide representative, authorized personnel from the departments of health services, income maintenance, aging. . . . Indigent persons shall be placed on any waiting list for admission to a facility and shall be admitted to the facility as vacancies become available, in the same manner as self-pay applicants.

While a number of states have similarly tough legislation that appears to prevent discrimination against indigent as well as private-pay residents, the sad fact is that enforcement of these regulations is uneven, and many states simply have *no* regulations on this matter. A related problem is that some state governments just look the other way when it comes to the private-pay case. It might be something akin to a conspiracy between Robin Hood and the Sheriff of Nottingham: The state continues to provide an unreasonably low reimbursement for the Medicaid beneficiary while allowing the nursing home to soak the private-pay residents through admissions donations and higher rates, which essentially are subsidizing the Medicaid recipients.

Here is an example of how admissions fees are solicited. Mr. W. is a fifty-year-old engineer whose mother needs care in a 150-bed, not-for-profit, skilled-nursing facility. He calls the nursing home and is invited to visit with Mrs. S., the chief social worker. At this initial interview, he is asked who will pay for his mother's care, which will cost approximately $100 per day, or $36,500 per year. Mr. W. says that his mother will pay for it herself. He is then asked whether he and/or his mother would be willing to sign a contract in which they agree to pay the private rate. He says yes. Mrs. S. asks Mr. W. to fill out an application and tells him that there is quite a long waiting list but that he should be hearing from the admissions committee within several days. He is also told that the committee, consisting of five members of the nursing home's board of trustees, has the final say on admissions to the home. About three days later, Mr. W. receives a call from Mr. X., who is an attorney and chairman of the admissions committee. Mr. X. asks Mr. W. to come to his downtown office and chat with him about his mother's application. At Mr. X.'s office, the first few minutes are cordial enough, mostly small talk about the excellence of the home and its fine reputation in the community. Next Mr. X. swings into action and tells Mr. W. about the long waiting list—perhaps he pulls out the list, showing him that his mother's name is at the bottom. Then Mr. X. discusses the dire financial straits of the home: "Last year we lost $150,000 because we want to provide your mother and everyone else's elderly parent a place where they can finish out their years with excellent care and dignity. But to do that costs real money. Mr. W., the fact is that each year we admit fifty new residents and only ten of those are not on Medicaid. Those ten new residents must share the burden of covering the deficit."

Mr. W., not quite comprehending what is happening, asks Mr. X. what he means about sharing the burden. The committee chairman replies that if you divide the $150,000 deficit by ten, that means each new private admittee should be willing to donate $15,000 to the home. Mr. W. asks if this is a requirement for admission and is told it is not. Mr. X. then reminds Mr. W. of the home's excellence and the long list. Not being too politic, Mr. W. asks whether a donation would expedite his mother's chances of being admitted sooner. Mr. X. says that admissions is a complicated business and the committee has considerable discretion, but he wouldn't want to suggest that a donation would guarantee swifter admission. He again assures Mr. W. that his mother will definitely be admitted sometime in the near future—as soon as the waiting list is cleared. Mr. W. finally takes the hint and shifts the discussion to the donation. First he asks whether $7,500 would be an adequate gift. Mr. X. says he is sorry, but they really need $15,000 for the deficit. Then Mr. W. asks if he can make it in installments of $5,000 a year for three years. Mr. X., a smart fund-raiser, knows when you have a donor, you had better get the money up front, so he answers negatively. Finally, Mr. W. asks, "What if I give you the money and my mother doesn't like the home after a few days or a week? Do I get it back? Or what if my mother dies the next day? Can I have the $15,000 returned?" "No," says Mr. X., "it is a no-strings, up-front cash gift to the building fund." The next day, Mr. W. delivers the "gift" to the nursing home, and to the amazement of all, a bed opens up for a person with the exact condition his mother is suffering from and she is admitted to the home—with slightly less financial baggage.

What I have described is most likely to happen in the not-for-profit homes that accept Medicaid residents as well as private-pay residents. Whether the donation is to a building fund or to the general operating budget of the home, the home's directors usually have a sense of the moral correctness of what the home is doing—that is, having the rich subsidize the poor—with the implication, although not the direct, unambiguous statement, that the donation will expedite a person's admission.

States such as Connecticut have effectively outlawed such preadmission solicitations. New York also appears to prohibit such behavior by a nursing home. In fact, New York went a step further in 1986 when it ran a "sting" operation against several New York City nursing homes, eventually indicting three top executives of two of New York's best homes. In that case, the homes had solicited a total of $55,000 from families of potential Medicaid beneficiaries, and thus had violated a 1982 New York statute. Eventually the administrators pleaded guilty to a lesser charge and the homes donated food to the elderly poor in lieu of a fine.

In summary, while government has winked at the admissions-fee fund-raising activity associated with private-pay residents, it is quite unlikely that any level of government will allow nursing homes to engage in such behavior toward those without financial assets.

DIFFERENTIAL RATES (AND ROOMS) FOR PRIVATE-PAY RESIDENTS

While charges for Medicare and Medicaid recipients are negotiated between the nursing home and the various governmental agencies, many states do not regulate the private-pay rates. This lack of regulation can result in higher rates for the private residents, and sometimes there is a difference in accommodations—with the private pay residents living in a newer wing or in the private rooms.

Once again, such discrimination based on source of payment may be effectively mitigated by a law such as Connecticut's, which, if fairly administered, would require treatment on a first-come, first-served basis; or more directly by Minnesota's law, which sets private rates in nursing homes at the exact level of the Medicaid rate.

For the record, I should note that I do not object to the practice of charging differential rates for private and Medicaid residents. Many states have a tendency to underpay nursing homes for Medicaid recipients, forcing the homes to cut corners or make up the difference in some other way, such as with higher private rates. Until the states follow Minnesota's lead of providing a Medicaid reimbursement that accurately reflects the costs of running the nursing home and allows a fair return on the equity in the home, then the only, and perhaps unfortunate, course of action is the present "Robin Hood" approach.

Many states do allow homes to charge differing private-pay rates according to the details of the room; for example, there are frequently differing rates for one-, two-, and four-bed rooms. Also, some homes charge rates that reflect whether the resident is in the newer, older, or redecorated part of the facility.

MEDICARE PAYMENT RESPONSIBILITY AGREEMENTS

Medicare coverage presents special problems for residents and their families because of the uncertainty of approval for claims. The typical process involves a resident being transferred from an acute-care hospital to a nursing home for Level I skilled-nursing services or perhaps rehabilitation care. Conferences held at the nursing home among the physician, the nursing staff, and the therapy staff will establish a plan of care for the resident. Then the documentation and the first round of bills are sent to Medicare. If everything appears acceptable to Medicare, the claim is approved, but sometimes Medicare does not approve the services. For example, there might be disagreement with the physician that the services are reasonable or necessary, or perhaps the services are not related to the prior hospital stay. Regardless of the reason for denial, the resident, if he or she cannot be switched over to the Medicaid program, will be responsible for the full cost of the services provided.

Unfortunately, a person might be in a nursing home for weeks before this determination is made by Medicare, and at that point the resident is likely to have run up a bill of several thousand dollars. Another related problem occurs when Medicare coverage expires for a beneficiary, usually when the allowable days have been used up. In such a case, if there is a need to keep the person in a nursing home, there are only two options—coverage by Medicaid and private payment.

PAYMENT IN ADVANCE

Here, too, states vary in what they will allow, but if a person is to be a private-pay resident, it is not unusual for a home to require a thirty- or sixty-day advance payment for room-and-board charges.

APPLICATION FEES

Very few homes charge a fee to apply for admission, and when it is charged, it usually is in the neighborhood of $25 to $75. The stated purpose of such a fee is to cover the costs of processing the application. An unstated purpose is to separate the applicants who are serious from those who are casually shopping.

PERSONAL-CARE EXPENSES

While the basic nursing-home charges cover the cost of room, board, and nursing services for a resident, there are numerous additional charges that homes can levy. However, what charges are permissible depends on the resident's pay status, with differing rules usually applying to Medicaid, Medicare, or private-pay residents.

For the Medicaid beneficiary, there are likely to be extra charges for such amenities as a television set, telephone service, and beauty parlor or barbershop visits. (These visits should not be confused with the periodic hair trims, shaves, or shampoos that usually are required as part of an individual's personal care.)

A home also might legitimately charge for any items that are special-ordered for a resident—for example, his or her favorite brand of toothpaste if it is not the brand the home normally uses.

For the Medicare beneficiary, Part A covers the basic room-and-board charges as well as the routine costs for nursing care and supplies. Part B covers diagnostic testing, physical and occupational therapy, and prescription drugs. Not covered by Medicare are the personal amenity expenses.

Although Part B may cover many of the therapeutic and diagnostic costs for private-pay residents, they frequently wind up with a number of small additional charges that can mount up to several thousand dollars over a period of a year or two. For example, one nursing home in California has a three-page price list that it gives to new private-pay residents. Examples of additional charges include the following:

Absorption dressing	$ 8.44–39.57
Decubitus pad	53.04
Enema bag	2.80
Enema bucket	3.04
Facial tissue	.75
Exam glove	.74
Wheelchair cushion	8.22

In addition to these charges, which must be borne totally by the resident, there are a number of other charges for which Part B pays 80 percent and the resident must make a 20 percent copayment.

At the above-mentioned California home, the resident is responsible personally for his or her incontinence supplies, which can amount to between $50 and $150 per month for disposable diapers.

Personal-laundry charges are another item that varies from home to home, with some providing it as part of the basic fee and others charging from $10 to $20 a month for personal wash-and-wear laundry. Residents who want dry cleaning or any services of a special nature should expect to pay for them privately. Some homes handle the personal-laundry problem simply by requiring the family or guardian to take care of it. In a unique and interesting twist on the matter, a few homes, such as one I visited in Bethesda, Maryland, have installed washers and dryers—some free and some coin-operated—and allow residents and their families to use the machines.

MEDICAL EXPENSES

Most nursing-home residents are covered by Medicare Part B and have a portion of their doctors' bills handled by Medicare. Depending on the resident's clinical condition, other medical expenses such as physical and occupational therapy, drugs, and specialized clinical supplies also are covered by Medicare.

CHARGES, COST, AND QUALITY

In nursing homes there is not always a perfect correlation among charges (what the resident is billed), cost of care, and quality. Indeed, many of the finest nursing homes I visited charged less than poorer-quality facilities but made up the difference through extensive fund-raising and income from endowments. In those types of facilities, the resident was essentially subsidized by the home's fund-raising activities.

As far as direct resident charges are concerned, it is fortunate when a nursing home has a clear charge structure that can be compared easily with those of other homes. More often, though, it will be necessary first to identify all of the services the resident is likely to require and then to ascertain the charges associated with those services. Only then will it be possible to compare rates. For example, many homes have an all-inclusive charge that may at first appear to be higher than rates charged by homes that essentially offer "unbundled" or à la carte rates. The true total can only be determined by adding all the expenses of the necessary ancillary services to the room-and-board rate.

While selection on the basis of price may be necessary in some instances, the issue of quality is of paramount importance for many people. Quality of care in nursing homes is a crucial and often confusing issue. For many families and residents, quality often is associated with the cleanliness or physical surroundings of the home. Without minimizing the importance of a nice environment, it is important to note that many nursing homes are truly selling "sizzle and not steak." They often play on children's guilt about putting a parent in a nursing home and allow these children to assuage that guilt by providing an environment with ersatz Chippendale furniture and a grand piano in a 1,000-square-foot living room. Of course, the reality is that residents cannot routinely use that living room for a host of reasons, such as lack of supervision or staff fear about soiled furniture from incontinent residents. A thoughtful purchaser of nursing-home care must look beyond these superficial aspects of quality. The next chapter begins the discussion of quality with an overview of the basic issues and an evaluation of some indicators and pseudo-indicators of quality care.

SIX

QUALITY:
The Elusive Search

They need a lot of love.

—K. G., *fifteen-year-old nursing-home volunteer*

A few years ago, I met with the health commissioner of a large industrial state, and one of the topics of our conversation was the quality of the several hundred nursing homes in his state. While neither of us had visited all of the state's homes, we both had seen enough of them to agree that many presented problems in terms of quality of care. Our observations were very much in line with those presented by a number of congressional investigatory committees, the U.S. General Accounting Office, and countless newspaper reporters aspiring to Pulitzer Prizes. Whether the information surfaced in newspaper exposés, congressional hearings, or carefully designed government research projects, the bottom line was always the same: A significant percentage of the nation's nursing homes deliver substandard care to their residents.

Since the commissioner and I both understood the reality, I asked him what he intended to do about improving the quality of the facilities in his state. The response I received was rather like a question I might pose to graduate students in a health-policy seminar: How does the state simultaneously meet its various goals, which are apparently in conflict—that is, how does it improve the quality of care in nursing homes while holding or cutting reimbursement to these homes and also ensuring that the stock of nursing-home beds in the state does not shrink but rather expands?

While this book is not about the public-policy problems in

nursing-home regulation, the health commissioner's dilemma does have an impact on what a consumer can expect in terms of government supervision of the industry. Indeed, when the small army of state inspectors go out to check the nursing homes, they are quite aware that while they can rough up the homes a bit, there are limits on how aggressively they can enforce regulations. And, in most areas of the country, those limits exist because the states need the nursing homes more than the nursing homes need the states.

An individual consumer, however, simply does not have to worry about the quality of a state's 5,000 beds; rather, he or she needs to be concerned about the quality of care given in only one nursing home. Since quality is one of the most crucial concerns of prospective residents and their families, this chapter provides a broad overview of the issues that are important for understanding quality. Specifically, it begins by defining quality within the context of the life of a nursing-home resident. Next, with a focus on food, a distinction is drawn between quality of care and quality of life. This chapter also discusses the serious and, unfortunately, bad news about quality, and a careful reading of this section will alert consumers to what experts look for as the benchmarks of quality. Finally, the chapter concludes with a discussion of the roles played by governmental agencies and voluntary organizations in monitoring and enhancing quality of care.

DEFINING QUALITY

According to the many nursing-home residents that I interviewed during my travels, good indicators of quality are cleanliness of the home, friendliness and attentiveness of the staff, adequacy and tastiness of the food, and freedom from urine odors. In many ways, their concepts are accurate manifestations of what researchers have also concluded are the necessary ingredients of a good-quality home—adequate staffing and attention to the individual needs of each resident.

Dictionary definitions of quality usually only provide us with abstract synonyms such as *excellence, first rate*, or *superior*. In 1986, the Washington, DC–based Institute of Medicine issued an important report entitled *Improving the Quality of Care in Nursing Homes*. While this report never explicitly defined quality, it did provide important conceptual assistance by identifying what it considered to be the three major characteristics of an excellent nursing-home program:

1. A competently conducted, comprehensive assessment of each resident
2. Development of a treatment plan that integrates the contributions of all the relevent nursing-home staff, based on assessment findings
3. Properly coordinated, competent, and conscientious execution of all aspects of the treatment plan

In order to qualify on all three of the attributes set up by the Institute of Medicine, a home would have to be staffed with well-qualified practitioners, it would need to create a work environment in which people were well motivated, and it would need to provide the physical and managerial resources to effect the program.

For a 1988 text, *Nursing Home Exemplars of Quality*, three people—one university-based, one from the Illinois state welfare department, and a third from a provider organization—teamed up for a research project on high-quality nursing homes in the state of Illinois. Their search for what they characterized as the unsung heroes of a frequently maligned industry yielded eight nursing homes but did not really move us closer to a definition of quality of care. However, the examples cited by the authors reflected adequate resources, a commitment to something more than profits, interested and active leadership and management, and caring staffs.

Perhaps most interesting is the authors' final observation that while the "run-of-the-mill" nursing homes offer poor-quality care, a number of other homes, acting under the same fiscal and regulatory constraints, offer quality care. This excellence, they suggest

. . . begins with a basic commitment to quality. As we have shown, in every first-rate home commitment goes hand-in-hand with a philosophy which sets the tone and defines the

priorities. These homes then put together a cohesive management team which embodies that commitment, and single-
mindedly translates it into the daily routine of nursing home
life.

DISTINGUISHING QUALITY OF CARE FROM QUALITY OF LIFE

Food service is a good way of illustrating the difference between quality of care and quality of life in a nursing home. As
is probably obvious, nursing-home residents are in many
senses prisoners of the kitchen and the institution. Usually
they are not in good enough shape to go out, and even if they
are, there may be no easily accessible restaurant. Indeed, considering the scores of places I visited, precious few were located in a neighborhood where a resident could even stroll
down to a corner grocery for a snack.

From a quality-of-care perspective, the first issue for concern is: **Has the new nursing-home resident's diet been properly selected, based on an adequate evaluation by a physician
or geriatric nurse practitioner and a dietitian?** A related
quality-of-care issue is whether or not there is periodic follow-
up on the nutritional status of the resident—that is, once a diet
has been established, is the resident reevaluated at periodic
intervals to ascertain how he or she is doing with it? For
example, the diet of a resident who has diabetes or high blood
pressure should be monitored and perhaps modified as the
resident's health status changes.

A second quality-of-care question is: **Is the food being
served in terms of adequate nutritional value?** For example,
is the resident receiving a sufficient amount of calories, and do
those calories come from the appropriate food groups?

Other quality-of-care issues exist behind the scenes in the
kitchen and storage rooms. For example, the quality of care
can be undermined by poor sanitation in the kitchen or by
food-service employees whose carelessness about personal hygiene transmits diseases to the residents.

However, all of these and many other quality-of-care issues

must stand in contrast to the quality-of-life issues that revolve around food. The nursing home interested in quality of life as well as quality of care recognizes the importance of food in the life of a resident. Such a home, while acknowledging the ever-present limits of institutional cooking and therapeutic diets, also recognizes that meal times for residents are as important for socializing as for eating. Such a home therefore approaches food as something more than merely fuel for the body. A few illustrations demonstrate how a nursing home can use food to enhance the quality of life for its residents.

At the Seattle Keiro Home, residents find Japanese foods on the menu at least once a day, and many traditional Japanese condiments are served with the western dishes. For example, while the usual breakfast might include toast, eggs, or cereal, several times a week breakfast at Keiro consists of miso soup, rice, toasted seaweed, or Japanese pickled plums. Lunches range from the western macaroni-and-cheese or meat loaf to fish teriyaki and various tofu dishes. Dinners tend to be mostly Japanese beef dishes or sushi.

Encouraging family and friends to share a meal with residents is a policy at the privately owned Ridge Terrace Health Center in Lantana, Florida. Here there is a weekly steak night when guests eat for $5—even better than the typical South Florida "early-bird" specials.

A dignified and pleasant place to eat meals is another positive quality-of-life factor. A mile or so from where I live in Northampton, Massachusetts, is the Pioneer Valley Nursing Home, a proprietary facility owned by a small regional chain that adds an unusual dimension to food service. Walking into the home's carpeted dining room with wood paneling, wall sconces, and chandeliers is like visiting the dining room of a fine hotel. Orders are taken from a selective menu by waiters and waitresses, checked in the kitchen for dietary appropriateness, and then delivered to the table. During one of my several visits, I was told that at one time there was even a maître d' for the evening meal.

Perhaps one of the most interesting approaches to deinstitutionalizing (or perhaps demystifying) food service in a nursing home occurs at St. Joseph's Manor in Portland, Maine. In that facility, one of the kitchen's interior walls has large picture windows so that curious residents can watch the preparation of the day's meals.

Cookouts, ice cream parties, theme parties, and special-occasion dinners—such as on Easter, Thanksgiving, Christmas, or religious occasions such as the Passover Seder—are very important for a nursing-home resident's well-being. If nothing else, they break up the monotony of eating 1,095 meals per year in the same place.

In trying to sort out what a visitor sees on an inspection tour, it is important to remember that we must look at the issues of both quality of care and quality of life. A glitzy dining room and no attention to a resident's dietary needs will be more damaging than a good, sound nutritional program and a modest dining room. The ideal is somewhere in between.

THE BAD NEWS ABOUT QUALITY

In 1974, Mary Adelaide Mendelson wrote a superb exposé of the American nursing-home industry appropriately titled *Tender Loving Greed*. The research for her book involved studying the specific nursing-home problems of Cleveland, Ohio, as well as visiting some 200 nursing homes throughout the country. Mendelson's pessimistic conclusion: "All over the country, nursing homes are similar, and similarly bad. Excellent homes are rare, and most of those that are considered good are good only by comparison to the majority that are worse." Indeed, of the 200 homes she visited, Mendelson rated only one as a good home. What apparently impressed her about that home was the honesty of the staff in admitting their shortcomings and attempting to rectify problems.

A few years later, in 1977, *Too Old, Too Sick, Too Bad* was published. Jointly written by former U.S. Senator Frank Moss and Val Halamandaris, a staff member of the Senate Special Committee on Aging, this volume synthesized thirty congressional hearings held between 1969 and 1976 on abuses in the nursing-home industry. As a catalog of nursing-home horrors, this book takes the prize. Using the thousands of pages of testimony Congress received, the authors present a vivid picture of resident abuse, disgusting and unsafe homes, and profiteering owners. At one point they note that "over 50 percent of the nursing homes are substandard."

While Moss and Halamandaris's estimate of 50 percent was based on their analysis of testimony to their committee, other estimates based on empirical research have also been offered. For example, in 1987 the U.S. General Accounting Office (GAO) issued a report to Congress based on an analysis of Medicaid and Medicare inspections over a four-year period. The first goal of the project was to determine the extent to which nursing homes repeatedly did not comply with federal and state regulations that might affect patient health and safety. A second goal, formulated by analyzing data from five states, was to "evaluate the adequacy of federal and state enforcement actions to correct reported deficiencies."

Based on its review of national data, the GAO reached a conclusion that was not very different from that of Moss and Halamandaris:

> Forty-one percent of skilled nursing facilities and 34 percent of intermediate care facilities nationwide were out of compliance during three consecutive inspections with one or more of the 126 skilled or 72 intermediate care facility requirements considered by experts to be most likely to affect patient health and safety.

Of greater concern, though, is what the GAO learned from its in-depth analysis of the inspection records of twenty-six problem-ridden nursing homes in Arkansas, California, Connecticut, Kansas, and Wisconsin:

> The 26 nursing homes were selected primarily on the basis of multiple repeat deficiencies. Among the most frequently cited deficiencies were inadequate nursing services, poorly maintained and dirty interior surfaces such as walls and floors, malfunctioning or broken plumbing, uncontrolled odors, improper use of physical restraints, and improper diets.

The report goes on to note that despite numerous deficiencies, most of the homes were recertified, and two of the three that in fact were decertified—that is, were no longer eligible for Medicaid or Medicare funding—were readmitted to those funding programs within seventy-six days. Indeed, the GAO noted:

> Facilities with deficiencies that do not seriously threaten residents' health and safety have continued participation in the programs for long periods without maintaining compliance with requirements. For example, a Kansas nursing home was cited in three consecutive inspections for having unqualified personnel insert or withdraw tubes used to administer drugs or provide nourishment, storing foods improperly, and failing to control facility odors, and in two inspections for failing to keep the building interior clean and well maintained. The nursing home received no penalty for the repeat deficiencies because termination was the only sanction authorized under Medicare and Medicaid.

In December 1988, the U.S. Department of Health and Human Services (HHS) threw another ingredient into the quality-of-care pot by releasing a seventy-five-volume state-by-state guide to nursing homes. With much fanfare, the departmental spokespersons explained that within these volumes consumers could find three-page summaries of the annual federal survey reports on each home. These reports, it was explained, rated each of 15,000 nursing homes on thirty-two separate health, safety, and care standards. Overall, the federal report painted a bleak picture of nursing homes: 29 percent of the skilled-nursing homes did not administer drugs according to the written orders of attending physicians; 11 percent of the nursing homes failed to meet basic housekeeping standards; 43 percent failed the standards for storing and preparing food under sanitary conditions; approximately 25 percent did not use proper isolation techniques to prevent the spread of infectious diseases; almost 30 percent were cited for failing to maintain the standard of personal cleanliness of residents; and another 25 percent were cited for not properly caring for the skin of residents.

The response to the HHS report was predictable. The nursing-home industry chided the government for releasing confusing and outdated information; academics said that the data were difficult to interpret; and nursing-home reformers said that the situation was worse than the report suggested. Senator John Heinz of Pennsylvania, whose Senate Select Committee on Aging had requested the GAO report—which was based on an analysis of 126 performance indicators, compared with the thirty-two used in the 1988 HHS report—summarized the burden felt by many when he stated, "Families in search of quality nursing care may be frustrated, if not out and out misguided, by the data as presented in this report."

INDICATORS AND PSEUDO-INDICATORS OF QUALITY

The scandals, exposés, and even government reports make it appear that there simply are *no* adequate nursing homes. This is not the case: There are numerous excellent homes with first-rate staff, programs, and facilities. The challenge is first to understand what the indicators of quality are in a nursing home and then to begin an investigation in pursuit of one bed in the right home.

For the remainder of this chapter, I shall discuss a number of indicators of quality. In the next chapter, I shall discuss specific indicators that represent standards for Medicare and Medicaid certification and that experts agree are of paramount importance in determining quality. These standards allow consumers to develop an individual assessment strategy for evaluating a particular nursing home.

INDICATOR 1: Licensure of the Nursing Home

Do not even bother with nursing homes that are not state-licensed! It is likely that such places are being run without anything close to minimal staffing levels, and there is a good chance that the buildings themselves violate fire, health, and safety standards that are basic safeguards of human life.

On the other hand, do not assume that state licensure is equivalent to a state seal of approval. Rather, think of licensure as nothing more than a basic registration that a nursing home obtains after meeting specified minimal qualifications. Consider the analogy of a driver's license—unfortunately, many people who should not be on the road have these licenses!

Licensure does tell you that a home is bound by a range of rules and regulations with mandatory standards in such areas as sanitation, health, safety, and (as noted in chapter 1) staffing. What licensure does not indicate is whether the facility is in violation of any of the standards and what the nursing home is doing to correct the violations. Further, since licensure enforcement tends to be a problem in many states, it is important not to stop at this most basic of indicators.

INDICATOR 2: Gold Stars

Some state governments, such as Kentucky and Texas, seem to operate with the idea that they can induce nursing homes to behave in a more responsible manner if they provide the homes with incentives to behave in the "right" way. One of these incentives is to offer a home gold stars or some variant on that award—such as a designation of "superior"—if it will meet additionally designated standards. For example, to get a superior rating in Kentucky, a nursing home must offer residents a number of designated "extras" that range from air-conditioning in all areas to establishment of a residents' council that selects weekly activities to a pet-therapy program. But what counts in this rating scheme can vary, with pet therapy as an example. Some homes merely have birds and goldfish present, while the program at Four Courts Nursing Home in Louisville include twice-monthly visits by a nationally certified pet therapist. Homes of varying quality strive for these ratings because of a desire to provide excellent care but also because of the market appeal of being identified in the "top" category—a category into which 65 percent of Kentucky's nursing homes fell.

While finding a five-star place is clearly to be encouraged, this designation should not be regarded as an undisputed stamp of high quality. Rather, it is a statement that a home's owners and managers have organized their facility so that they can obtain the stars or designation. Sometimes what has to be done to attain the special designation is essentially meaning-less, while at other times it does indeed represent a commit-ment to quality.

To evaluate accurately the importance of these special des-ignations, it is necessary to contact the agency issuing the awards and find out what the standards are for the various designations; how those standards are evaluated; and, finally, how many facilities in the state meet those standards. If every nursing home in a state can meet the standards for gold stars, one might conclude that the standards are too low or that the state is the paradise of nursing homes.

INDICATOR 3: Licensure of Administrator

This is one of the most meaningless of indicators. For reasons that are not entirely clear to me, numerous pamphlets and other nursing-home guidebooks suggest that one indicator of quality is the licensure status of the nursing-home adminis-trator. The reality is that for a facility to operate in most states and to be certified for Medicaid or Medicare, the administra-tor must be licensed.

Perhaps of greater importance is the relative ease of passing the licensure examination to become a nursing-home admin-istrator. Once an administrator is licensed in one state, it is quite simple to obtain reciprocity in other states as well as to renew the license by attending continuing-education courses. Also, since the owners of private nursing homes, or the boards of not-for-profit homes, do not have to be licensed unless they actually function as the home's administrator, it is likely that the person who is the licensed administrator, particularly in a home operated as a for-profit corporation, may not have the major say in the policy and management of the home. Rather, the person pulling the strings may be an unlicensed owner who is not involved in the day-to-day operations of the home.

INDICATOR 4: Medicare and Medicaid Certification

Not every nursing home in the country is certified by Medi-care or Medicaid. Some of these uncertified homes, such as Presbyterian Village in Dallas, appear to provide excellent care and meet most of the federal and state standards for certification. The decision of these homes not to be certified by these programs usually is based on economics—that is, the homes are interested primarily in catering to a totally private-pay clientele, and their market position allows them to do so without the constraints that governmental certification would impose upon them.

To be certified for Medicare and/or Medicaid, the nursing home must go through annual state inspections and meet hundreds of requirements that are focused on the structure of the home and the procedures it follows. The assumption behind the certification system is that a home will be better for its residents if it is properly structured—for example, if it has the correct policies and staffing in place and it follows the correct procedures, such as for administering drugs to residents.

Unfortunately, even if the assumption is correct, there are major problems with the certification process. In its important 1986 study of the quality of care in nursing homes, the Institute of Medicine identified many of these problems:

> . . . the regulations do not require assessment of the quality of care being delivered; rather, they require assessment of the facility's structural capacity to provide care; the survey process emphasizes paper compliance rather than observation and interviews with nursing home residents; many of the standards are vague and depend too much on unguided judgments by surveyors, many of whom are untrained. Surveyor judgments are frequently inconsistent; what is deemed acceptable by one surveyor may be unacceptable to another.

In other sections of its report, the Institute of Medicine identified a wide range of problems with certification involving the state's role in managing the process and enforcing the standards.

The report went on to propose myriad reforms, including changes in staffing requirements for nursing homes, a mandatory training period for aides, and elimination of the distinction between skilled-nursing facilities and intermediate-care facilities.

However, the most important change in the assessment of

quality came in the nature of a new process for carrying out the mandated surveys. This new procedure, which was being developed before the Institute of Medicine report was issued, is the Patient Care and Services survey—commonly called the PaCS survey. In essence, it focuses less on the structural elements of an institution and more on patient care. (In chapter 7, the PaCs process is explained in more detail so that consumers can use its data in order to make an individual assessment of a home.)

INDICATOR 5: Organizational Memberships

Nursing homes, like most other business enterprises, frequently belong to a number of trade associations. Since membership in these organizations normally requires nothing more than payment of dues or perhaps endorsement of a vague set of ethical precepts, such membership is essentially meaningless in terms of being a guarantee of quality.

The fact that a nursing home is a member of the Chamber of Commerce, the Better Business Bureau, the United Way, the American Health Care Association (the trade organization of for-profit homes), or the American Association of Homes for Aging (the trade association of the not-for-profit nursing homes) should be of no consequence in the decision to select or reject a particular home. This does not suggest that such organizations do not provide a valuable function but rather that membership in them simply is not an indicator of quality.

INDICATOR 6: Accreditation Status

Accreditation is a horse of a slightly different color, since it is handled by the Joint Commission on Accreditation of Healthcare Organizations, the same organization that accredits hospitals. For nursing homes, accreditation is a voluntary process that involves a home's being inspected during a several-day period by a team of outside experts who compare the activities within the home to a set of externally developed standards.

As with the licensure process the reviewers are looking primarily at the structure of the organization and the processes within it. Presently, accreditation of nursing homes tends to answer the question, "*Can* this organization provide quality health care?" What the accreditation process does *not* tell us is the answer to a different question: "*Does* this organization provide quality health care?"

While the commission should be applauded for its diligent work on shifting accreditation from a process-and-structure orientation to one that focuses more on quality of care and outcomes, the reality is that accreditation status currently is of limited value to the consumer. Some nursing-home administrators I interviewed indicated that it was not particularly difficult to become accredited and that they simply used accreditation for marketing purposes. Even if these comments are accepted at face value, accreditation nonetheless indicates that a home is voluntarily opening itself to review by outsiders—and that, in and of itself, is positive.

In sum, if a home is accredited, it is a plus factor but not necessarily the ultimate statement of excellence. On the other hand, a home should not be viewed as unacceptable merely because it is *not* accredited by the commission. Indeed, some of the best homes I have seen are not accredited.

INDICATOR 7: Teaching Affiliations

Nursing-home teaching affiliations come in a variety of guises. The premier affiliations are those with medical schools and teaching hospitals. The Monroe County Hospital in Rochester, New York, which is really a several-hundred-bed skilled-nursing facility, is an example of what can be possible under the right circumstances. During the time when Franklin K. Williams, M.D., directed this institution, prior to his departure for Washington to head the National Institute of Aging, the facility developed a reputation for excellence. This excellence was doubtless due to his leadership and the home's affiliation with the University of Rochester, which managed the facility and based some of its medical-school faculty there. The result of such an affiliation is the traditional commitment of a medical school or teaching hospital to quality, plus increased visibility and the scrutiny of the facility by a professional public vitally concerned with quality. Dr. Williams pointed out to me that the teaching nursing home has three advantages for its residents: (1) The resident is likely to find a higher quality of professional staffing because of the affiliation; (2) the presence of students who "are eager and often have the time and availability to care" is a big bonus; and (3) the teaching milieu often results in higher standards for the nursing-home's management.

Other less intense but important affiliations are the type one sees at the Shalom Geriatric Center in Kansas City, Missouri. Through the efforts of Dr. Frederick Franklin Holmes, who is the Edward Hashinger Distinguished Professor of Medicine and Gerontology at the University of Kansas Medical Center, and Mel Weissman, Shalom's executive director, a program was established in which medical students would do a thirty-day rotation through the nursing home, which meant that six to eight senior medical students would spend three afternoons per week for a month at the home doing admissions and annual physicals. In addition, the nursing home and the medical center jointly established a medical fellowship in gerontology and have jointly sponsored research and educational programs.

Regardless of the specifics of an affiliation between a nursing home and a medical school or teaching hospital, it appears that any such arrangement has a positive outcome for the quality of the services in the home.

A number of nursing homes also have teaching affiliations with programs for training nurses, aides, technicians, therapists, social workers, and administrators. Generally, these programs reflect positively on the home, but they should not be considered major statements of a commitment to quality. The reason for this is simple: Most of the teaching programs focus on the educational experience of the student and simply do not delve into the job of evaluating or influencing the quality of care in an institution.

CONCLUSION

Finding a nursing home that offers quality care is not an easy task. The nursing homes themselves, which frequently sell style and not substance, do not make the task any easier. And, as various studies and reports demonstrate, the government does not make the task any easier, either.

In the end, it is the consumer who must separate the wheat from the chaff. To do this effectively requires research, knowledge, and effort. This process begins in the next chapter with an example of the three-page summary of a nursing home's evaluation, which is available for homes throughout the country.

SAMPLE NURSING-HOME–ADMISSIONS APPLICATION

APPLICATION TO
Four Courts, Inc.

Name _____
Admit Level of Care _____
_____ Permanent
_____ Temporary

2100 Millvale Road
Louisville, Kentucky

1. Name _____ Age _____
   _{Last}   First   Middle/Maiden
2. Present Address _____
3. Former Addresses (Most recent first)
   _____ From _____ To _____
   _____ From _____ To _____
   _____ From _____ To _____
4. Date of Birth _____ Place of Birth _____
5. Marital Status: _____ Married _____ Single _____ Widow _____ Separated _____
6. Occupation _____ Last Employed _____
7. Social Security Number _____ Medicare Number _____
8. Reason(s) for requesting service: (Please check one or more)
   ☐ (a) Family unwilling or unable to keep applicant
   ☐ (b) Applicant cannot continue alone
   ☐ (c) Applicant unhappy in present environment
   ☐ (d) Present arrangement too expensive for applicant or family
   ☐ (e) Other (Specify) _____
9. Additional pertinent information about present circumstances and need for Home (add any specific information
   to clarify reasons given under #8).
10. Medical:
    (a) Name of your physician _____ Alternate Phys. _____
        Address _____
    (b) Date of your last medical examination _____
    (c) Have you been hospitalized within the last five years? _____
        Where _____ Date _____
        Where _____ Date _____
    (d) Have you been a resident of any other Home for Aged, Nursing Home or Institution? _____
        Where _____ Date _____
    (e) Have you applied for admission to another Home or Institution? _____
        Where _____ Date _____
    (f) Dentist _____
        Phone # _____ Last Exam _____
    (g) Podiatrist _____
        Phone # _____ Last Exam _____
    (h) Optometrist/Ophthalmologist _____
        Phone # _____ Last Exam _____
11. What is your general health? (insert "Yes" or "No" for all items)
    _____ (a) Take Care of self completely
    _____ (b) Need some help in dressing, eating, walking, etc. (underline or specify) _____
    _____ (c) Chronically ill (Underline or specify) Diabetes, heart, other _____
    _____ (d) Partially bedridden
    _____ (o) Completely bedridden
    _____ (f) Wheelchair case
    _____ (g) Other conditions, such as blind, deaf, etc. (Please state) _____
    _____ (h) Mental condition (Underline) Excellent, Fair, Poor, Forgetful, Other _____
    _____ (i) Able to travel: without help _____ with help _____ (If no, explain) _____

Four Courts, Inc.

2100 Millvale Road
Louisville, KY
40205-1699
1-502-451-0990

12. Do you have any income at present? ☐ Amount $ _____ per _____
13. Check source of income:
   ☐ Children   Amount $ _____   ☐ Social Security   Amount $ _____
   ☐ Pension   Amount $ _____   ☐ Old Age Assistance   Amount $ _____
   ☐ Own Funds   Amount $ _____
   Other (specify) Source _____ Amount $ _____
14. (a) Have you any money in banks at present? _____
        Name of Bank   Address   Book No.   Balance

    (b) Did you ever have a bank account? _____
    Name of Bank _____ Address _____ Book No. _____ Date Closed _____
15. Have you a safe deposit box? _____ Where? _____
    Where did you last have a safe deposit box? _____ When? _____
16. Have you cash on hand? _____ If so how much? $ _____
17. Name of person holding funds for you.
    1. Name _____ Address _____
    2. Name _____ Address _____
18. Other resources (Check and give information to identify specifically)
   ____ Real Estate 1. _____   ☐ Stocks
               2. _____   ☐ Jewelry
   ☐ Mortgages _____   ☐ Furniture
   ☐ Bonds _____   ☐ Other
19. Have you during the past five years disposed of money, insurance, real estate, securities, personal property? ____

(Yes or No)

If Yes   What   To Whom   When

20. Have you any life insurance? (Check)   Yes _____   No _____
Company   Policy No.   Type Policy   Date Issued   Amount   Premium Paid By

HOSPITALIZATION AND MEDICAL BENEFIT COVERAGE

21. Are you covered ....Yes _____ No _____
   ☐ Blue Cross Group # _____ Certificate # _____ Plan _____
   ☐ Blue Shield Group # _____ Certificate # _____ Plan _____
   ☐ Other _____ Certificate # _____ Plan _____
   ☐ Medicaid # _____
22. Religion _____ Rabbi/Minister _____ Phone # _____
   Would you like us to notify at admission? ☐ Yes   ☐ No
23. What is your funeral home preference? _____
24. Have you reserved a grave? _____ Where? _____
   Who holds the deed? _____
25. Persons to be notified in case of emergency:
      Name   Address   Phone #   Relationship

Four Courts, Inc.

2100 Millvale Road
Louisville, KY
40205-1699
1-502-451-0990

1. STATEMENT OF ACKNOWLEDGEMENT

In compliance with Federal Regulations, we must have a signed record stating that you received a copy of the Facility's Patient Rights, a copy of "Access and Visitation Rights," and that you understand the rights presented therein. Also, that you have had explained to you the various charges for care provided by Four Courts. We/I sign this acknowledgement with the understanding that the Patient Rights benefit the patient's interest and individuality; and further that they have been explained to me orally and that I have received a copy for my future reference. Also, the charges associated with the costs of providing care have been explained orally and a copy given to me. I have no further questions with regard to the rights of patients in this facility.

2. AUTHORIZATION TO REQUEST PAYMENT

I hereby authorize the staff doctors of Four Courts, Inc., to request payment under part B of the Medicare Program for services rendered to me. This authorization will remain effective until such time as the undersigned is no longer a resident of Four Courts.

3. AUTHORIZATION TO RELEASE/SECURE INFORMATION

I hereby authorize Four Courts, Inc., to release any information concerning my medical history and/or treatment to persons in need of such information and who are properly authorized. I hereby authorize Four Courts, Inc., to secure information concerning my medical history and/or treatment, laboratory reports, any information pertinent to my care received from any physician or health care facility I might have used, so as to provide me with the care needed.

4. CERTIFICATION OF INFORMATION

I certify that the information given to me in applying for payment under Title XVIII of the Social Security Act is correct. I authorize release of any information needed to act on this request. I request that payment of authorized benefits be made in my behalf.

5. BED RESERVATION

Should my family member, _____ , be out of the facility for any reason, I understand that I must assume financial responsibility during the period of absence from Four Courts if I want his/her bed reserved. I further understand that if I don't reserve the bed, the room will be assigned to a new patient currently on the waiting list.

6. AUTHORIZATION TO MANAGE RESIDENT'S ACCOUNT

I, _____ do/do not authorize Four Courts, Inc., to manage a
    (Resident's Name or Responsible Party)

resident's account for _____ . I understand that this account will be maintained in accordance with standard 249.12 (a) (1) (iii) of the state regulations. I also understand that a quarterly statement of account will be given to me in accordance with all government regulations showing all deposits and withdrawals from this account.

7. AUTHORIZATION TO ADMINISTER T.B. TEST

I do/do not give my permission to administer a T.B. test to _____
annually, according to State Regulations. A chest x-ray will be done if T.B. test is refused.

NAME OF PATIENT (Please Print) _____

PATIENT'S SIGNATURE X_____

WITNESS SIGNATURE X_____

RESPONSIBLE PARTY'S SIGNATURE X_____

WITNESS SIGNATURE X_____

DATE _____

❧

Four Courts, Inc.

2100 Millvale Road
Louisville, KY
40205-1699
1-502-451-0990

AFFIDAVIT:

I hereby apply for admission to Four Courts. If admitted, I agree to comply and conform to its rules and regulations and its Constitution and By-Laws, as the same may be constituted and exist from time to time. I understand that if admitted, I am to remain at the Home only as long as my stay is agreeable both to the Home and to me. Either of us have the absolute right to terminate my residence at any time, for any reason satisfactory to either of us. I know that the Home does not make agreements for life care.

I agree that, during my residence in the Home, I shall pay to the Home its monthly charge for my maintenance. I understand that this charge may be altered in the discretion of the Home, for any reason. Billing is prepared per month.

I understand that although I shall be primarily responsible for the payment of such charge or charges, such indebtedness shall be a charge upon my estate, and a statement in writing signed by the Executive Director of the Home (or his agent, appointed in writing), as to the amount of such monthly charges due or past due shall be conclusive and binding upon my legal representatives as to the amount and reasonableness of such charges.

If I and/or my family are not financially able to meet the full monthly charge, I agree to apply for public assistance and to abide by the Commonwealth's regulations in regard to such aid.

I also agree that this application shall be subject to the approval of the medical and administrative staff of the Home.

And I agree to execute and deliver such further agreement or agreements or other instruments as may be requested to effectuate my admission.

I warrant the statements and answers given to me in this application to be full and complete, and also certify that I have truthfully answered all questions.

Witnessed by:

1. _____ _____
   (Name & Address)   (Applicant's signature)

2. _____ _____
   (Name & Address)   (Date)

As responsible agent, _____ I hereby
                      (Specify Relationship to Applicant)

attest to and am responsible for the terms stated in the above affidavit and its agreements.

Signed _____

Address _____

Date _____

Witnessed by:

1. _____
   (Name & Address)

2. _____
   (Name & Address)

The following authorizations must also be signed to complete application requirements.

In behalf of _____
             (Insert Applicant's Name)

I also hereby expressly authorize and request: –

(a) Any and all insurance companies in which I am insured, or which hold funds of mine or payable to me, and

(b) Any and all banks and bankers which now hold or heretofore held funds of mine, and

(c) Any person, firm or corporation which holds funds of mine or payable to me

(d) Any social agencies to whom I am or have been known

(e) Any doctors, hospitals, and clinics to whom I am or have been known

to give full and detailed information regarding the same to Four Courts or its accredited representatives.

Witnessed by:

1. _____ _____
   (Name & Address)   (Signature of Applicant or Responsible Agent)

2. _____ _____
   (Name & Address)   (Date)

SAMPLE NURSING-HOME–ADMISSIONS APPLICATION

THE MEADOWGREEN

Last Name		First Name					Middle Initial	
Previous Address	City		State	Zip	Sex	Marital Status	Social Security Number	
Age	Birth Date	Birth Place			Citizen of		Military Service	
Name of Husband or Maiden Name of Wife				Address Phone			Birth Place	
Guardian or Closest Relative		Relation		Address			Phone	
Financial Guarantor				Address			Phone	
Notify in Case of Emergency 1		Relationship		Address			Phone	
2								
3								
Church Preference		Name of Clergy		Address			Phone	
Name of Father		Birth Place		Maiden Name of Mother			Birth Place	
Admitted from		Referred By			Admission Date		AM PM	
Hospital Preference					Ambulance Preference			

Dentist	Address	Phone Office	Home
Attending Physician	Address	Phone Office	Home
Alternate Physician	Address	Phone Office	Home
Funeral Home	Address	Phone Office	Home

Pharmacy Preferred

Health Insurance Benefit Number (Medi Care No.)	Hospital Insurance
Burial Insurance	

Admitting Diagnosis _____

Authorization is hereby granted to summon any licensed physician in an emergency and release such information as may be necessary.

     Signed: _____

STANDARD ADMISSION WAIVER

The undersigned hereby requests the admission of _____ to your Home and upon such admission agrees to pay cost of patient's ca giving due allowance for Alternate Assistance, if any. As further consideration of such admission, it is mutually agreed that said Home shall not be held liable for accide of injury to patient during residence. It is further agreed that management shall not be responsible for money or valuables left in possession of said patient whil resident of this Home. Management, however, agrees to exercise ordinary care in maintenance of patient's clothing, but assumes no responsibility for wear and tea same. Undersigned represents that he is patient's _____ and has legal authority or consent of patient to so act in his or her behalf.

Witness	Date	Signature
Date Readmitted	Physician	Diagnosis
Date Readmitted	Physician	Diagnosis

❧

SEVEN

FINDING THE RIGHT NURSING HOME:
Identifying and Evaluating the Options

Caveat Emptor
(Let the Buyer Beware)

Some interesting analogies exist between the processes of selecting a nursing home and selecting a college or a job. For example, the governing principle for college selection in my family was that we could go anywhere we received a scholarship—or, alternatively, anywhere that the New York City transit system could take us on a token and a transfer. This simple approach limited choices and made the decision relatively easy.

Today it appears that, despite the enormous cost of a college education, tens of thousands of high school students and their families are taking a broader and more aggressive approach to finding the right college. They start identifying possibilities by speaking with friends, acquaintances, school-based counselors, and high-priced consultants. Next the student and the family peruse college catalogs, as well as the videotapes and laser disks that colleges mail to prospective applicants. While both star athletes and star scholars can expect everything from letters to invitations for free trips to distant campuses, in the more typical case, a parent winds up traveling with a high school junior or senior from city to city, campus to campus, and admissions office to admissions office. Eventually, they will have visited a number of campuses; taken tours; talked to students, administrators, and perhaps faculty; and formed impressions about the colleges. Finally, they select a small number of schools for application, and, from those that accept the student, they choose one for matriculation.

The processes of finding the right job and the right community are equally time-consuming. Someone searching for a new position usually has to pursue countless leads, submit résumés to scores of companies, and interview at dozens of firms before finding the right one. Then the second part of the equation comes into play: Is it the right community? People frequently select or reject jobs for such factors as the cost of living in a community, housing, taxes, and the quality of the elementary or secondary education. In my own case, I turned down one excellent job offer because the commute (after I tested it on two occasions) would have been horrendous and another because, after checking with local environmentalist groups, I learned that the city's water and air were heavily polluted and not likely to be cleaned up for a decade.

Finding the right nursing home is equally complex. For most people, the process is akin to moving into a new home in a new community—two steps that no one would undertake in a cavalier manner. Indeed, it is important to reemphasize here that going into a nursing home is not like going into a hospital, where patients are whirled through a revolving door before anyone knows his or her name. A new nursing-home resident is the new kid on the block in a small, tightly knit community of several hundred people, some of whom reside in the community twenty-four hours a day, others of whom work in the community eight hours a day. The search for the right nursing home is hard work. It requires learning about those who reside in the nursing home; about those who attend to the needs of the residents; and about those who manage, control, and implement the policies and procedures of the home.

SELECTING A LOCATION

A friend recently asked my advice about a nursing home for his mother, who still lived in his hometown of Philadelphia. I responded, assuming he was asking about homes in our part of New England, but I was wrong. He wanted to know about options in Philadelphia, because, as he explained, his mother's connections were there and his brother still lived in a neigh-

boring community. I provided several names in the Philadelphia area but also suggested that he and his family consider
the Massachusetts options I had first identified. Apparently
my counsel had an impact, because several days later, he ap-
proached me for more information about the Massachusetts
homes.

This vignette illustrates two of the most common reasons
people appear to select a particular location: current residence
and proximity to family. Current residence is a powerful force
because it seems to minimize the separation from a familiar
environment. Those who move into a local nursing home are
likely to find themselves among former acquaintances or perhaps classmates. Because they are locals, they can easily continue some of their community activities and interests, which
would be disrupted with a move to a more distant location.
George T., a ninety-one-year-old widower who recently
passed away, illustrates my point. Until his last days, despite
being confined to a wheelchair, he remained active in his Masonic lodge, going to weekly meetings and other outings via
transportation provided by the nursing home and the Masons.

Also, it should be reiterated that a significant percentage of
nursing-home residents wind up in a long-term-care facility
after a hospitalization (with that hospitalization most often
occurring in the local community). The job of the discharge
planner, as noted in chapter 2, is to place the hospital patient
in an acceptable nursing home as quickly as possible. In general, the discharge planner is working with a number of local
nursing homes for this purpose and is not focusing on a long-
term stay. Unfortunately, once a person is in a particular
nursing home, a transfer to a second home is highly unlikely.
The term that social workers and researchers use for this situation is *transfer trauma*—that is, the trauma of transferring is
so great that elderly people, once they have adjusted to a
facility, simply do not wish to move even if the next home
would be significantly better. This point was emphasized for
me in one city where I visited a nursing home that was superb
in every respect except that it had a fifteen-month waiting list.
In a neighboring city, I visited one of the most crowded,
shabby, and poorly staffed homes that I have ever seen. Here

I learned that many of the residents in this third-rate home had been on the waiting list for the first home but had chosen not to go there when space became available for them. It appeared that the residents and their families had made their adjustment to this unsatisfactory place and did not want to go through the difficulties of a second move.

The other major reason for selecting a particular location is the proximity of close relatives, usually children. Moving close to children may come with the cost of severing long-term neighborly relationships, but it does have the benefit of ensuring family contact. The M. family, for example, decided to move both the mother and the father, who lived in suburban Chicago, into a nursing home several hundred miles from the Windy City but within a two-hour drive of three of the four children and a twenty-five-minute drive of one child. The parents, who had been active church members, found a hospitable environment in their new home, which was operated by their same denomination. In commenting on this new arrangement, one of the M. children noted that after years of confusion and racing back home every time one of the parents became ill, there was a new orderliness and harmony in their relationship. Also, after years of worrying about phone calls in the night, they could finally sleep, knowing their parents were being cared for properly in an excellent institution.

Each family needs to work out its own solution, clarifying which location would be in the best interests of all parties. However, it is important to recognize that there are options in terms of locations, and while some homes are geographically restrictive in terms of the catchment area they will serve, many are willing to consider applicants from anywhere in the country, particularly if that applicant has a local connection.

MAKING A LIST AND CHECKING IT TWICE

There are a number of different ways to develop an initial list of nursing homes once the location has been selected.

The simplest—and, in my judgment, least helpful—way is to use the Yellow Pages of your telephone book. The list there is normally comprehensive and accurate with regard to address and phone number, but it is altogether too easy to be drawn to those homes that have invested in extensive display advertisements and to overlook much better places that do not choose to market themselves through the directory. Indeed, I looked through the Yellow Pages in a dozen cities where I knew of at least one excellent facility, and in each instance, the excellent home did not advertise. Further confounding the difficulty of using the telephone directory is finding the proper name of a nursing home. For instance, in one city I found a nursing home listed under its popular and not its corporate name; in another city I found that nursing homes were listed under the legal/corporate and not popular names.

A second and more useful approach is to go to a local library and review any nursing-home directories they may have. Frequently, a state department of health, aging, or welfare has compiled a guidebook that provides basic information on nursing homes. Thousands of libraries have in their reference sections a book published by the Phoenix, Arizona–based Oryx Press: the *Directory of Nursing Homes* (3rd edition, 1988). This volume contains entries on almost 17,000 nursing homes, and the information generally covers size, ownership, staffing, and facilities. However, since the directory facts come from a variety of sources, including the facilities themselves, they may not always be totally complete or accurate. In cross-checking the entries of a number of excellent homes with which I am familiar, I found that they tended to provide minimal information. At $195 per copy, the book is too costly for an individual to purchase, but it is worth seeking out at the library. It can be a valuable tool for establishing a preliminary list.

A third way of developing a list of potential homes is through personal or professional referrals. Local physicians, social workers, and members of the clergy frequently can identify possible facilities. Occasionally a family member may even have had experience with a local nursing home.

The next method is to use official state agencies. In Appendix 1 are lists of state long-term-care ombudsmen, offices of elder affairs, and state health departments. Each of these offices will identify possible homes in an area, but you should not expect much more from them. Generally speaking, I have found state employees quite reluctant to disclose anything other than the most basic information about a nursing home.

If you are committed to seeking a not-for-profit nursing home, contact the state affiliate of the American Association of Homes for the Aging (see Appendix 1), or, if there is no affiliate in your state, contact the national headquarters at 1129 20th Street, NW, Washington, DC 20036, (202) 296-5960. If you call, ask for membership services.

A second group with information about privately owned (for-profit) nursing homes is the American Health Care Association, (see Appendix 1).

USING THE PaCS SURVEY TO CULL THE LIST

This task was made dramatically easier in December 1988 when the Health Care Financing Administration (HCFA) of the U.S. Department of Health and Human Services released its seventy-five-volume *Medicare/Medicaid Nursing Home Information* report designed to help consumers make informed judgments on nursing homes. These reports, which include three pages of summarized information on every Medicare- and Medicaid-certified nursing home in the United States, are available in the various state Medicare and Medicaid offices, most state health and welfare offices, the offices of congressmen, Administration on Aging offices, and, probably in the future, in libraries and the offices of nursing-home ombudsmen. The data presented in these reports provide a useful starting point for any investigation of a nursing home. The remainder of this chapter shows how such data can best be used.

In order to explain these three-page summaries, the next section of this chapter describes the Patient Care and Services (PaCS) survey, which gave rise to the federal reports. Following this description is a copy of an actual summary of an institution, and the last section has some final comments on the value of these reports in terms of culling the list of potential homes.

The PaCS Survey—How the Pros Evaluate
Nursing Homes

In the mid-1980s, in response to myriad criticisms of the Medicaid and Medicare survey process, the federal government developed a new approach to inspecting nursing homes and qualifying them for governmental reimbursement—the so-called Patient Care and Services survey, known in the trade as the PaCS survey. Its basic idea is that each year qualified state inspectors will, without advance notice, survey each nursing home in their state and evaluate the home's performance against a set of standardized criteria. In the past, evaluation tended to focus on the structure of the home and its ability to deliver the necessary care. The PaCS survey has shifted the focus to the actual delivery of care, which is investigated by records review, observation, and interviews with staff and residents.

In practice, the PaCS survey has several sections, but the first two—which address the institution's compliance with life safety code and structural requirements (such as whether the home has qualified staff or an effective disaster plan)—are essentially similar to the pre-PaCS surveys. Several features are new and important about the PaCS approach, however. The first of these is attitudinal. Surveyors are told that the surveys are an inspection and enforcement process and that their role is to "assess the quality of care provided by the health care facility," which means checking that the nursing home's activities are in compliance with federal regulations. Indeed, surveyors are specifically cautioned against providing any technical advice or consultation to the nursing homes.

The second major change is the survey itself, which is divided into seven tasks that the inspectors are expected to complete: (1) entrance conference; (2) in-depth, integrated tour of the facility with a selected sample of residents for subsequent follow-up; (3) observation, interview, medical-record review of each sampled resident; (4) drug pass observation; (5) dining-area and eating-assistance observation; (6) deficiency-statement formulation; and (7) exit conference. This new process compels the surveyors to carefully examine outcomes in a nursing home. For example, in their instructional manual, surveyors are told that their in-depth integrated tour is supposed to last approximately three hours, and during it, they are required to focus on the resident-care areas, the types and patterns of care delivered in the nursing home, and the general physical environment. For example, during an inspection of one home that I visited, the inspectors found a number of problems during their tour, including a clogged lint trap in a clothes dryer, greasy and dirty exhausts over a stove, frozen food that was not labeled, and an improperly disposed-of contaminated dressing. The manual also states:

> Each resident should be scanned for the following while touring:
>
> - Personal hygiene, grooming, and appropriate dress
> - Position
> - Assistive devices
> - Ambulation
> - Other restorative devices
> - Restraints
> - Rehabilitation issues
> - Hydration and nutrition status
> - Infection control
> - Resident rights
> - Activity for time of day (appropriate or inappropriate)
> - Emotional status
> - Level of orientation
> - Awareness of surroundings
> - Behaviors
> - Cleanliness of immediate environment (wheelchair, bed, bedside table, etc.)
> - Odors
> - Adequate clothing and care supplies, as well as maintenance and cleanliness of same

Surveyors are also urged to observe the nature of interactions between residents and staff members. If a home has a resident council, its president and other officers are supposed to meet with the inspectors. Finally, as part of this task, the surveyors select a sample of residents, approximately 10 percent, for a personal interview as well as an in-depth record review. Later in the process, staff members also are interviewed.

At a later point in the survey, the inspectors observe a "drug pass," which means they examine the process of dispensing medications to approximately twenty residents in the home. Since a prime concern in nursing homes is medication error, the surveyors are most often evaluating whether the proper drugs are being given in the proper manner. The final part of the survey involves direct observation and occurs in the dining areas, where the inspectors watch the serving of at least two meals to ensure that the right diets are being delivered to the right residents. Other items the surveyors are trained to look at include "staff interaction with residents, prompt and appropriate assistance, adaptive equipment usage and availability, as well as dress and hygiene appropriate for meals."

What results from these tours, interviews, structured observations, and records reviews is a report that identifies whether or not the facility has met the hundreds of standards demanded for Medicaid or Medicare participation. The nursing home must then take corrective action on any deficiencies or risk loss of funding or, in some cases, closure.

Overall, these surveys normally involve two inspectors, at least one of whom is a nurse. In addition, the teams frequently are supplemented for short periods by specialists in areas such as dietetics or pharmaceuticals. Federal regulations suggest that the typical survey should take a total of about sixty person-hours, which, based on my own observation, is about par for the course. For example, in one survey I observed at a 200-bed home, the team of two nurses arrived unannounced the day before Thanksgiving and stayed through the following Tuesday. This core group of two nurses put in a total of four days each (sixty-four hours), plus, on one day, two associates also put in a full day, for a grand total of eighty hours.

The report reviewed in the case study that follows was generated by the PaCS process as outlined. The actual report the surveyors and the nursing homes use is significantly different from the report presented here and those in HCFA's *Medicare/Medicaid Nursing Home Information*. The final report deals with hundreds of standards and considerably more commentary than is found in these three-page summaries.

In describing the limitations of these summaries, the Health Care Financing Administration makes five important points. First, it notes that the data for these reports were generated from the work of more than 3,000 surveyors who each made individual judgments about the particular homes' deficiencies. In essence, there is an important acknowledgment that the survey process, despite aspirations toward great objectivity, has a significant subjective element within it.

Second, the survey process itself ensures only that a nursing home has met the minimal federal standards to participate in the federal financing programs. There is no attempt within the process to separate the outstanding home from the merely acceptable home. Obviously, the surveyors, who visit dozens of homes each year, are likely to be quite insightful about the strengths and weaknesses of the homes in a region. Unfortunately, though, they do not share these insights with the general public, and we are left with only the results of their work—merely a report card that tells whether or not an individual home passed the qualifying test.

Third, the summary only provides information on whether or not a particular home has met thirty-two important standards. Nothing in the summary speaks to the several hundred other federal standards a home must meet. However, a simple remedy is at hand. You can call the state licensing authority for nursing homes (see Appendix 1) and order the full inspection report—and also the latest one—for the home(s) you are interested in considering. If you are fortunate enough to live in California or one of the other states that require homes to post their latest reports on easily accessible consumer bulletin boards, you will only have to walk in their front door in order to read the reports.

A fourth limitation is again related to the process, which is a several-day survey once every twelve to fifteen months. How a home behaves on a certain day with junior Inspector Clouseaus looking into every nook and cranny may not be an accurate reflection of its functioning throughout the year. Further, even if it is, staff or managerial changes in the period between the inspections can dramatically alter what goes on in a home, but it takes years before such changes are reflected in reports.

A related problem is that the published summaries inevitably are out of date, and there is a good chance that even the latest full report you order from the state health or welfare agency will also be out of date.

Finally, the summary tells nothing about the gravity of a deficiency, whether the deficiency is continuing, or what the home did about remedying the problem.

On the other hand, the report does present an easily accessible point for starting one's research into a nursing home.

CASE STUDY: Green Valley Nursing Home

Each survey report is divided into three sections. The first section provides superficial identifying information about the home, the second provides basic information about the residents of the home, and the last section—"Selected Performance Indicators"—provides data about deficiencies from the PaCS survey in thirty-two areas.

Street Address:		City and State:	
736 GREEN VALLEY AVENUE		GREEN VALLEY, OREGON	
Participation:	# of Beds:	Type of Ownership	Survey Date:
MEDICARE/ MEDICAID SNF/ICF	200	NON-PROFIT OTHER	09/22/87

SELECTED RESIDENT CHARACTERISTICS

Total Residents on Day of Survey: 194	Medicare Residents: 0	Medicaid Residents: 150

Caution: A large number of residents with these characteristics does not indicate whether those residents are receiving appropriate or inappropriate care. It may reflect the facility's ability to provide highly specialized care and services.	FACILITY		STATE	NATION
	#	%	%	%
Bathing Residents requiring some or total assistance in bathing.	166	85.6	78.2	81.5
Dressing Residents requiring some or total assistance in dressing.	158	81.4	82.0	83.2
Toileting Residents requiring some or total assistance in toileting.	119	61.3	70.4	73.8
Transferring Residents requiring some or total assistance moving from bed to chair or to tub or toilet.	137	70.6	80.6	77.2
Continence Residents with catheters or partial or total loss of bowel or bladder control.	112	57.7	70.5	68.2
Residents on individually written bowel and bladder retraining program.	11	5.7	6.1	4.6
Eating Residents receiving tube feedings or requiring assistance with eating.	50	25.8	34.6	37.7
Completely bedfast residents.	1	0.5	1.9	3.4
Residents confined to chairs.	55	28.4	41.4	50.8
Residents requiring restraints.	53	27.3	41.2	41.3
Confused or disoriented residents.	121	62.4	58.8	58.4
Residents with bed sores.	0	0.0	5.2	7.1
Residents receiving special skin care.	109	56.2	40.4	31.2

SELECTED PERFORMANCE INDICATORS

"Facility" column indicates deficiencies found at the time of survey. The Federal Government requires facilities to correct deficiencies immediately or to submit a plan indicating deficiencies will be corrected within a reasonable period of time. "State" and "Nation" columns indicate number and percentage of occurrence of deficiencies in other facilities in the State and Nation. "Met" means that the facility is in compliance with the specific requirement. "Not Met" means the facility was deficient in the indicated area at the time of the survey.

Reminder: These 32 selected performance indicators do not represent all the requirements a facility must meet. There are over 500 separate requirements. The information presented below does not reflect the severity or the duration of the problems leading to a deficiency. A deficiency may represent an ongoing problem or a one-time failure of a single staff person.	FACILITY MET/ NOT MET	NUMBER & PERCENT OF FACILITIES NOT MEETING REQUIREMENTS			
		STATE		NATION	
		#	%	#	%
The facility ensures that its written procedures regarding the rights and responsibilities of residents are followed.	MET	2	0.6	201	2.1
The facility uses a system that assures full and complete accounting of residents' personal funds. An accounting report is made to each resident in a skilled nursing facility every three months.	MET	35	10.7	518	5.5
Each resident is free from mental and physical abuse.	MET	5	1.5	168	1.8
Drugs to control behavior and physical restraints are only used when authorized by a physician in writing for a specified period of time or in emergencies.	MET	8	2.4	806	8.5
Each resident is given privacy during treatment and care of personal needs.	MET	47	14.4	1618	17.1
Each resident is allowed to communicate, associate and meet privately with individuals of his/her choice unless this infringes upon the rights of another resident.	MET	0	0.0	36	0.4
Each resident is allowed to retain and use his/her personal possessions and clothing as space permits.	MET	1	0.3	205	2.2

Except in a medical emergency, a resident is not transferred or discharged, nor is treatment changed radically, without consultation with the resident or, if the resident is incompetent, without prior notification of next of kin or sponsor.	MET	2	0.6	30	0.3
The facility ensures that the health care of each resident is under the continuing supervision of a physician.	MET	9	2.8	145	1.5
Emergency services from a physician are available and provided to each resident who requires emergency care.	MET	3	0.9	49	0.5
Nursing services are provided at all times to meet the needs of residents.	MET	15	4.6	508	5.4
Each resident receives daily personal hygiene as needed to assure cleanliness, good skin care, good grooming, and oral hygiene taking into account individual preferences. Residents are encouraged to take care of their own self care needs.	MET	62	19.0	2816	29.8
Each resident receives care necessary to prevent skin breakdown.	MET	46	14.1	1733	18.3
Each resident with a bed sore receives care necessary to promote the healing of the bed sore including proper dressing.	MET	37	11.3	1052	11.1
Each resident who has problems with bowel and bladder control is provided with care necessary to encourage self-control, including frequent toileting and opportunities for rehabilitative training.	MET	26	8.0	1512	16.0
Each resident with a urinary catheter receives proper routine care, including periodic evaluation.	MET	46	14.1	1665	17.6

❧

SELECTED PERFORMANCE INDICATORS

Reminder: These 32 selected performance indicators do not represent all the requirements a facility must meet. There are over 500 separate requirements. The information presented below does not reflect the severity or the duration of the problems leading to a deficiency. A deficiency may represent an ongoing problem or a one-time failure of a single staff person.	FACILITY MET/ NOT MET	NUMBER & PERCENT OF FACILITIES NOT MEETING REQUIREMENTS			
		STATE		NATION	
		#	%	#	%
Each resident received proper care for injections (shots), fluids supplied through tubes, colostomy/ileostomy, respiratory (breathing) and tracheotomy care, suctioning and tube feeding.	MET	35	10.7	1123	11.9
Each resident receives rehabilitative nursing care to promote maximum physical functioning to prevent loss of ability to walk or move freely, deformities and paralysis.	NOT MET	30	9.2	2045	21.6
Each resident needing assistance in eating or drinking is provided prompt assistance. Specific self-help devices are available when necessary.	MET	46	14.1	1662	17.6
Drugs are administered according to the written orders of the attending physician.	MET	93	28.4	2739	29.0
Menus are planned and followed to meet the nutritional needs of each resident in accordance with physicians' orders, and to the extent medically possible, based on the recommended dietary allowances of the Food and Nutrition Board of the National Research Council, National Academy of Sciences.	MET	17	5.2	1389	14.7
Therapy is provided according to orders of the attending physician in accordance with accepted professional practices by qualified therapists or qualified assistants.	NOT MET	27	8.3	587	6.2
Services are provided to meet the residents' social and emotional needs by the facility or by referral to an appropriate social agency.	MET	12	3.7	816	8.6

An ongoing program of meaningful activities is provided, based on identified needs and interests of each resident. It is designed to promote opportunities for engaging in normal pursuits, including religious activities of the resident's choice, if any.	MET	23	7.0	1099	11.6
Appropriate staff develop and implement a written health care plan for each resident according to the instructions of the attending physician.	MET	26	8.0	1270	13.4
Toilet and bath facilities are clean, sanitary, and free of odors.	MET	55	16.8	1216	12.9
All common resident areas are clean, sanitary and free of odors.	NOT MET	71	21.7	1041	11.0
All essential mechanical and electrical equipment is maintained in safe operating condition.	MET	14	4.3	1413	14.9
Resident care equipment is clean and maintained in safe operating condition.	NOT MET	59	18.0	1408	14.9
Isolation techniques to prevent the spread of infection are followed by all personnel.	MET	64	19.6	2340	24.7
The facility has available at all times a quantity of linen essential for proper care and comfort of residents.	MET	17	5.2	700	7.4
Food is stored, refrigerated, prepared, distributed, and served under sanitary conditions.	NOT MET	130	39.8	4050	42.8
Reminder: The results of the full survey are available from the State survey agency or the State ombudsman.					

The first section contains only the home's address, the total number of beds, a general statement of ownership, and the survey date. It is important to recognize that a great deal of information still is unknown, and it should be known in order to make an informed decision. For example, one learns nothing about the mix of beds in the home—that is, how many are authorized for skilled care and intermediate care—or the home's rates and services. Other important information not presented in this summary relates to staffing; type of facilities available, such as private or semiprivate rooms; programs at the nursing home; and admission requirements or restrictions.

The second section of this report provides data on selected resident characteristics. A review of the first six categories— bathing, dressing, toileting, transferring, continence, and eating—plus the other six characteristics, can provide a sense of the type of resident who lives in the home and can, on a superficial level, be used to compare resident populations from one facility to another.

However, these data also have limitations. To begin with, the first four categories of bathing, dressing, toileting, and transferring are listed by the percentage of residents who require some or total assistance. Obviously there is a broad range between "some" and "total." Continence has an equally broad spectrum, which includes everyone with catheters as well as those with problems ranging from partial to total loss of bowel or bladder control. In eating, the range goes from people receiving tube feedings to those requiring assistance.

The final six characteristics present a host of definitional problems. For example, what exactly does it mean that a resident requires restraints or that a resident is confused or disoriented? Also, regardless of how these terms are defined, it is important to remember that with the possible exception of "completely bedfast," all the other terms require someone's judgment for categorization. Further, within any one category there is no distinction between minor and major problems— such as minor, easily treatable bedsores and major recurrent bedsores.

In summary, while it is necessary to look at this first page of the report with a critical eye, particularly since this information comes from the nursing home itself and may not be completely verified by the inspectors, it does provide enough information for a preliminary idea about a home. For example, after reviewing the first page of the Green Valley report, I would be able to make a preliminary judgment about its location and infer that its residents probably were more active than residents in other homes in the area. These data also suggest that the home must be reasonably well staffed because of the activity associated with continence and toileting. Finally, the total absence of residents with bedsores and the significant activity in special skin care would also support my hypothesis of a well-staffed and aggressive nursing program.

Next comes the heart of the summary—the two-page documentation of thirty-two selected performance indicators. While it is unclear why the federal government decided to select these specific items from a field of some 500 possible standards, it does appear that all of these are valuable indicators of the quality of care and services in a particular home. But, as mentioned earlier, it is unfortunate that the data merely present conclusions—that is, whether a particular standard has or has not been met. When a standard has been met, nothing tells us whether the home is meeting that standard in a truly outstanding manner or merely an acceptable one. When a standard is found not to have been met, no further explanation is provided as to the problems in the home that led to the finding.

In the case of Green Valley Nursing Home, five of the standards on the third page of the form were considered "not met." In order to judge whether or not any of the hundreds of federal standards are met, the inspectors are provided with guidelines for observation, interviewing, record review, and factors for evaluation before rendering a decision. As an illustration of these guidelines, consider Green Valley's violation of the standard for cleanliness of the common areas. The language of the standard is that "All common resident areas are clean, sanitary, and free of odors." The guidelines advise the inspectors to "use senses—sight, hearing, olfactory—when surveying common areas such as lounges, lobby, corridors." The guidelines also instruct the inspectors to ask residents the following questions:

1. Do you think the corridors and lounges are usually clean?

2. Do they have unpleasant odors?

Finally, the inspectors are told that in evaluating their decision with regard to this standard, the factor to consider is: "Floors and furniture should appear clean—free of gross contamination."

By going back to the inspectors' observations on their original survey form, I learned that four findings led to Green Valley's failure to meet this standard:

1. Some shower stalls were covered with built-up soap scum;

2. Ceiling vents had a large accumulation of dust;

3. Horizontal surfaces such as moldings, window frames, and lighting fixtures had an accumulation of dust;

4. Encrusted food spills were found on seats of chairs and table pedestals.

What is perhaps of most importance to the discerning consumer is not the violation itself but rather why it occurred and what the institution did in response to it. In discussions with the administrator of Green Valley, I learned several things. First, the problem was not, in his judgment, as serious as the report makes it appear. The inspectors did what he called a "white glove" test and failed to recognize that some of the deficiencies they observed occurred because of the timing of their inspection. For example, showers are scrubbed down weekly and the inspection came immediately prior to a scrubdown. Regardless, he did acknowledge that a better cleaning schedule would alleviate almost all of these housekeeping problems, and after the inspection, the housekeeping and maintenance staff did develop new routines.

It is also important to notice whether deficiencies are corrected by the institution or recur in the next inspection. In the case of Green Valley, this unmet standard was not a problem at the next inspection. Among the facts *not* learned about Green Valley from this report are that it is located on well-landscaped property in a pleasant residential neighborhood; it has an excellent physical plant with many private rooms; its charges are quite competitive with those of neighboring nursing homes; it has a full-time medical director; and its staffing ratio is one of the highest in Oregon. Developing this kind of profile requires a personal interview, but it is necessary to sort out all of the preliminary data before that interview. To assist with this process, it is best to utilize the Worksheet for Selecting First-Round Homes (see below).

USING THE WORKSHEET FOR SELECTING FIRST-ROUND HOMES

The accompanying worksheet is designed to organize the basic material about a set of nursing homes in a comprehensive and orderly manner. By going through each of the sections of the worksheet, potential residents and their families will, before even visiting a particular home, be able to eliminate some names from their list if they find that these homes simply do not stack up well next to others. Even if you decide to visit all of the homes listed on the worksheet, the process of developing the information is quite useful as a way of "doing homework" beforehand.

The first part of the form asks for basic information about the facility. Question 4 is an important one but may require some work, including review of local maps, calling the nursing home, or obtaining information from various transit services. The concern being addressed here is that homes that are isolated tend to present problems in terms of visitors as well as in regard to activities and volunteer programs.

Part II asks for information about the size and potential mix of residents in the home. Occupancy rates and waiting lists also are important. For example, Connecticut's strong waiting-list law requires the home to admit residents based on date of application, so if a particular Connecticut home has a two-year wait and you need a bed within ten days, it may not be worthwhile to interview at such a packed facility. Item 5, which requires identification of the home's ownership and special auspices, is an important matter to clarify before a visit, since it is possible in some areas for a home to deny admission to people who are not affiliated with its ownership. I suggest finding out names, phone numbers, and in some instances length of service before a visit. Knowing the name and reputation of the medical director may also be useful in making a decision.

The financial information section will give comparable data for institutions and also will clarify what resources may be needed to enter a particular home. I suggest you summarize the HCFA data in part IV. By reviewing the different sections of the HCFA report and using your own words to fill in the information, you will begin to have a clearer picture of each home. The last section is for recording comments and impressions from others who have experienced the home or its staff. These remarks are useful when used in conjunction with all the other data.

All the data necessary for completing these forms can be obtained from the library resources mentioned earlier, the HCFA report, and a phone call or two to the nursing home.

Based on this information, the next step is to select homes for a preliminary visit. At the end of the worksheet is a section for recording your choices. There is also space for recording reasons. By taking the time to articulate the reasons, you also tend to clarify what is important and what is not. The next step is the preliminary visit, which is the focus of chapter 8.

Part I   Identifying Information

1. Name of Home _____
2. Address _____
   _____
3. Phone Number _____
4. Proximity to main roads/public transportation _____
   _____

Part II   Key Information

1. Number of Beds _____
   a. Number of private rooms _____ Semiprivate _____
   Other _____
2. Present occupancy _____ %
3. Waiting list _____
4. Number Skilled Beds _____ Number Intermediate Care _____
5. Ownership _____
   a. Religious or fraternal auspices _____
6. Name of Administrator _____
   Number of years at nursing home _____
7. Name of Director of Nursing _____
   Number of years at nursing home _____
8. Name of Medical Director _____
   Telephone Number _____
   Relationship to nursing home _____
9. Name of Social Services Director _____
   Relationship to nursing home _____
10. Names of other admissions personnel _____
    _____
11. Hospital affiliations _____

Part III.   Financial Information

1. Room charges: Private _____ ; Semiprivate _____ ;
   Other _____
2. Additional charges:

3. Application Fee _____
4. Medicare certified _____
5. Medicaid certified _____

Part IV: Summary of HCFA Report

1. Needs of the Residents:
   a. Apparent physical needs

   b. Apparent psychosocial needs

2. Unmet Performance Indicators

Part V: Recommendations/Neighbor, friends, family, clergy, doctor, etc.

Decision:
(   ) Visit   (   ) Do Not Visit   (   ) Put on hold

❧

EIGHT

THE PRELIMINARY NURSING-HOME VISIT

Having selected several possible nursing homes via the tasks described in chapter 7, your next step is to visit these homes. Analyses of the reports of the Health Care Financing Administration (HCFA) and other publications, as well as recommendations, are useful for narrowing the list of nursing-home candidates but they are no substitute for a personal inspection of the home. This chapter deals with a number of crucial questions, including why a preliminary visit is necessary, who should go, how to arrange for the visit, what to expect from the nursing home, whom to interview, what questions to ask, what to look for, and how to evaluate your findings.

PURPOSES OF THE PRELIMINARY VISIT

Just as a young physician cannot learn to be a surgeon simply by reading textbooks, it is impossible to learn about specific nursing homes without investing the time to visit them. The central purpose of this preliminary visit is to give a potential resident and his or her family a chance to decide whether a particular home is worth a second and more thorough look, but the visit also can serve a number of other objectives. Perhaps the most important objective is to clarify whether a nursing home is really the most reasonable alternative for a loved one. By seeing several nursing homes and carefully observing the facilities, staff, residents, and programs, and getting a sense of the rhythm of the day, everyone will be in a better position to understand the consequences of a move into a nursing home.

The preliminary visit is also an opportunity for clarifying such issues as the cost of the nursing-home care, the availability of private rooms or rooms for married couples, and the types of specialized programs set up for residents with dementia or Alzheimer's disease. The visit also provides an opportunity for developing skills in interviewing staff and residents and observing life in a nursing home. Finally, during the visit, you can obtain helpful material such as residents' handbooks, contracts, and annual reports if you did not receive them in advance.

THE PRELIMINARY-VISIT TEAM

It is best if more than one person makes the preliminary visits, and perhaps as many as three or four people should go. If possible, this group should include the prospective resident as well as some close friends or relatives. Frequently, the prospective resident is not available or is not well enough to make the trip, in which case a family may have to accept the responsibility for a visit.

There are two major reasons to send a team rather than one person: (1) With the team approach, no individual needs to take the entire responsibility for the decision or has to be the focus for negative feelings generated about a nursing-home placement; and (2) two heads are better than one. There is much to see on a visit, and two or more people are likely to observe more and have useful and complementary insights. The value of the team approach will become clear once the group has reconvened after the visit to share impressions of the home.

ARRANGING THE VISIT

Although Medicare/Medicaid inspectors make unannounced visits and the nursing home is obligated by law to respond to their demands, it is wise to make an appointment for a preliminary visit. Advance scheduling allows the home to arrange for the various interviews (suggested in the next section) and also to give the staff a chance to plan your visit when it is most convenient for them. The value of this is that you are an expected guest, and, if the home is properly responsive, you will not be rushed through the visit. While some might argue that advance notice provides the nursing home with a chance to put its best foot forward so you may not get an accurate picture of it, I do not put much weight on this position. Most nursing homes are busy places, and they simply do not have the time or resources to spiff up the premises for just one set of interviewers.

In planning for this preliminary visit, you should be prepared to answer several questions from the home about the prospective resident and perhaps about finances. Additionally, ask the home to make arrangements for your group to tour the facility, talk with some residents, and meet with the key members of the staff who will be responsible for delivering care to the future resident. The accompanying Preliminary-Visit Arrangement Checklist will help organize these aspects of a visit.

PRELIMINARY-VISIT–ARRANGEMENT CHECKLIST

Nursing Home Name _____

Phone Number _____

Directions to facility _____

Date of Visit _____

Part I [Have this information about the prospective resident ready before calling the home]

1. Name of prospective resident
2. Date of birth
3. General health status
   Any specific medical problems?
   Any mental health problems?
4. What type of help, if any, is needed for any of the following activities:
   Bathing
   Dressing
   Toileting
   Transferring (moving from bed to chair, tub, or toilet)
   Continence (bowel and bladder control)
   Eating
5. How will the cost of nursing home care be financed—private pay, insurance, Medicare, Medicaid?

Part II: [Visit plans]

1. Be prepared to tell the home who will be coming on the visit and their relationships to the prospective resident.
2. Be prepared with several alternative dates.
3. TELL the person arranging the visit that you would like to meet with the following people:
   a. The administrator
   b. The director of nursing
   c. The director of social services
   d. The activities director
4. TELL the home you also wish to meet with several residents— preferably ones who are about the same age and sex as your prospective resident.
5. TELL the home you wish to tour the facility and see a resident's room, the dining areas, the activities and therapy areas, and other commons areas.
6. ASK the home if it is possible for you to eat a meal there at your own expense.
7. ASK the home to send you a residents' handbook, contracts, annual report, or other public-relations documents prior to your visit.

THE INTERVIEWEES AND AREAS OF INQUIRY

The visit to the nursing home is primarily a series of interviews and observations. This section identifies those who should be interviewed, what questions should be asked of them, and why. The next section provides some suggestions concerning observations.

Interviewing the Administrator

The administrator is responsible for the day-to-day management of the nursing home and has a great deal of influence over the entire atmosphere of the institution. Some administrators keep themselves ensconced in their offices and learn about the home through written or oral reports delivered by subordinates. Others have adopted the "MBWA" approach—management by walking around. This second type of administrator tends to know every nook and cranny of the home and seems genuinely interested in the welfare of the residents. Indeed, touring a facility with such administrators is exhausting merely because they stop to greet each resident and their families. However, the exhaustion is well worth it when one recognizes that the caring atmosphere created by this kind of manager goes a long way toward deinstitutionalizing a nursing home.

The agenda for the meeting with the administrator has several elements. First, it is important to obtain background information on the administrator and, by extension, a sense of the commitment of the institution to top-notch administration. An institution committed to first-class management is likely to have an administrator who has a master's degree in some area of health administration, gerontology, human services administration, business administration, or social work. An alternative might be someone with a background in a technical and clinical specialty, such as nursing, physical therapy, or occupational therapy, plus training for nursing-home licensure. Finally, as in other fields, it is important not to be influenced solely by the presence or absence of a person's academic achievements—there are plenty of excellent nursing-home administrators who, through years of experience, have grown into the job and become models of excellence.

On the other hand, a warning flag should go up when an administrator's background and training seem inappropriate to the job. While the individual may indeed be quite competent, one must question the commitment of the owner or board that hires such a person. For example, I visited one home where the administrator had been an automobile salesperson for ten years before becoming an activities assistant and then activities director at a small nursing home. Armed with his four years of experience in activities and a new nursing-home license, he was able to obtain the job of administrator in another small nursing home. While it was clear that he was quite a nice person, and no doubt an excellent salesman for the nursing home, it was equally clear that he was merely a front man for the absentee-owner, who ran the home from the other end of a phone line. In my opinion, such people are hired by owners who need to meet the letter of the law—that is, a state requirement for an on-premises licensed administrator—but not the spirit of the law, which calls for a professionally trained independent administrator.

The administrator can be a source of considerable information about the facility, and the Administrator Questionnaire—Preliminary Visit (AQPV) should be used as the principal tool for gathering the necessary information about both the administrator and the institution.

The first group of questions focuses on the home's ownership and governance—who is truly in charge. As already noted, it is my judgment that organizational anatomy is destiny. In practice, this means that one can tell a great deal about the functioning of a home by learning about its ownership and how that ownership chooses to govern the home.

The second set of questions speaks to the background and qualifications of the administrator in order to plumb the commitment of the home to management excellence.

The third set of questions deals with several specific and critical issues. First, it is important for a prospective resident to be aware of the medical supervision of the facility. Most nursing homes contract with someone who has the title of medical director and spends very little time in the home, perhaps two to four hours a week. If the home is a skilled-nursing facility with a significant number of very elderly and sick people, several hours of medical supervision may be too meager. If the new nursing-home resident is likely to need more intense medical supervision, it is important to find a facility with a more extensive medical program.

In response to the question about medical supervision, you are most likely to learn that there is a very part-time medical director but that each resident has his or her private physician. This may sound good on paper, but the reality is that most nursing-home residents do not receive much attention from local practitioners, although obviously there are exceptions. The typical story is that the local doctor merely breezes through the home, making perfunctory visits. A related question is whether or not the home employs a geriatric nurse practitioner. Such specially trained nurses, functioning under a physician's supervision, can in many instances provide the necessary on-site medical care required in a nursing home.

The next issue relates to transfers. In the best of situations, a resident would not be moved to another nursing home except for specific clinical reasons or at the request of the resident for social reasons, such as being geographically closer to relatives. The major concern about transfers is economic— that is, does the home transfer people when they run out of private-pay funds? This problem is likely to occur primarily in the strictly private-pay home that is not Medicare- or Medicaid-certified. However, some of these homes, such as Presbyterian Village in Dallas, have policies that provide for "scholarships" to individuals who have been residents and have run out of funds.

The issue that should be explored next is that of any recent deficiencies on the regular Medicare/Medicaid survey. It will be useful to hear the administrator's explanation of why the deficiencies occurred and how the home acted to remedy them.

The last three questions ask the administrator to identify the strengths and weaknesses of the nursing home, to explain the home's philosophy, and to provide an example of how that philosophy is put into practice. While these questions tend to be open-ended, the answers may be very revealing in two ways: (1) They may provide you with an indication of the willingness of the administrator to be candid with you, and (2) they may reveal some possible areas for further investigation.

I. Ownership and Governance

A. Is this a <u>for-profit, not-for-profit,</u> or <u>government-owned</u> nursing home?

1. IF FOR-PROFIT:

a. Who owns this facility? Where are they located?

b. Is it part of a chain? If yes, how large a chain?

c. Are you [the administrator] one of the owners?

2. IF NOT-FOR-PROFIT:

a. Who is on the governing board of the nursing home?

b. How do people get on the home's governing board?

c. Does the home have a particular religious, fraternal, or other special orientation?

d. How often does the board meet? How often does the board's executive committee meet?

3. IF GOVERNMENT-OWNED:

a. What agency of government is responsible for the home?

b. Does the home have a supervisory or governing board?

c. Who serves on the board? How often does it meet?

II. Administrator's Education and Experience

a. How long have you been a licensed nursing-home administrator?

b. What is your educational background?

c. How long have you been at this nursing home? In what capacity?

d. What other experience have you had in nursing-home administration other than your present position?

III. Administrative Issues

a. Who is the nursing home's medical director? How much time per week does he or she spend at the home? Does the home employ a geriatric nurse practitioner?

b. What is the home's policy on transfers? How many people have been transferred to another home in the last year? What were the reasons for the transfers?

c. On the 19____ Medicaid/Medicare certification survey, the following deficiencies were noted: Please explain.

d. What do you see as the strengths of this nursing home?

e. What do you see as the weaknesses of this nursing home?

f. What is the philosophy of the nursing home? Can you provide an example of how that philosophy is put into practice?

❧

Interviewing the Nursing Director

The nursing director is a key person in the hierarchy of the nursing home. It is usually the responsibility of the nursing director to recruit and train staff, and the quality of her leadership (most are women) can have an important impact on the quality of care at the home. The interview with the nursing director should result in two types of data for your subsequent analysis: (1) data about the nursing director's personality and style, and (2) quantitative data about the nursing organization.

The interview ought to begin with a request for information about the director's experience and education. Although these two items are important, I should note that one of the most sensitive and thoughtful nursing directors I met in my travels was a man who was only two years out of nursing school. Although a neophyte in the world of nursing, he had chosen it as a second career after more than a decade as a successful middle manager in a national corporation. In this individual's case, his skills in management and his commitment to the elderly clearly outweighed his inexperience in nursing.

The next questions are crucial for clarifying the home's nursing picture. The first three questions ask for staffing numbers, with the third question being the most important: How many nursing hours per resident per day does the home provide? While there is no "right" answer, it appears that the better homes try to reach a figure in excess of 3.0, and some get up to 3.5. If you hear numbers much higher than 3.5, the person providing the information probably does not know how to calculate the ratio. When that occurs, do your own calculation by dividing the number of residents into the number of available nursing hours in the day (this includes all nursing staff—RNs, LPNs, and LVNs, and aides).

The next few questions ask about nursing vacancies, turnover, wages, and pools. In response to questions about the number of staff in a nursing home, nursing directors often have told me how many authorized positions they have, not how many are on staff. Vacant positions do not provide nursing care. These questions clarify the stability of the home's staff and the competitiveness of the home in recruiting nurses from a marketplace with a chronic shortage. The question about pools may be of particular importance. Pool nurses are essentially day workers who fill in when a home has an unanticipated staff shortfall. In the best of situations, pool nurses are used rarely. However, pool nurses are a reality, and the better nursing homes have organized a pool from which to call in nurses who are familiar with the home's routines and can easily jump into the operation. Any home that appears to be excessively dependent on pool nurses should trigger a warning flag.

The last two questions under nursing department issues focus on nursing unit assignments and the transfer process. The answers to these questions will indicate the sensitivity of the home to the needs of the residents and give some indicator about the likely future relationship among the home, the resident, and the family. Fundamentally, these questions plumb the issue of whether that relationship is consultative and participatory or autocratic, perhaps dictatorial.

The final set of questions begins with an inquiry into the nature of special care units at the home and then focuses on nursing deficiencies that may have been reported on the Medicare/Medicaid survey form. By frankly presenting this information, you as an interviewer have an opportunity to clarify any apparent problems with nursing and also to evaluate how the home responds to criticism.

The last two questions appear on each of the questionnaires because if several people from the home respond independently to these questions, you as the interviewer eventually will be able to patch together a clear picture of strengths and weaknesses.

I. Director's Education and Experience

    a. How long have you been director of nursing? What other nursing positions have you held?

    b. What is your educational background?

II. Nursing Department Issues

    a. How many full-time or full-time-equivalent RNs do you have at the home?

    b. How many full-time or full-time-equivalent other licensed nurses do you have at the home?

    c. How many nursing hours per resident per day does the home provide?

    d. How many nursing vacancies presently exist?

    e. How much turnover do you experience each year in the nursing department?

    f. What are the starting wages for RNs, LPNs/LVNs, and aides?

    g. Are nursing staff permanently assigned to particular units or do they routinely rotate?

    h. Are pool nurses heavily relied on?

    i. What is the process for assigning new residents to a particular unit?

    j. Once on a particular unit, are residents ever shifted to other units? If yes, what is the transfer process and to what extent is the resident involved in the decision? Is the family involved in the decision?

III. The Home in General

    a. Does the home have special care units such as an Alzheimer's unit? How does the special care unit(s) differ from the general care unit(s)?

    b. On the 19____ Medicaid/Medicare survey report, the following deficiencies were noted in nursing: Could you please explain what happened to cause these deficiencies and how they were corrected?

    c. What do you see as the strengths of the home?

    d. What do you see as the weaknesses of the home?

❧

Interviewing the Social-Services Director

As with the questionnaire for the nursing director, the first group of questions provides background information concerning the director, and data reflecting the home's commitment to the social-service function. The second set of questions elicits what type of support can be expected from the social-work staff for residents and their families. Of particular importance in this section is the fourth question, which asks about anticipated adjustment problems and how the social-services department helps ease this transition. Since the move into a nursing home is traumatic for all parties, it is helpful to have a home that is sensitive to this issue and experienced in dealing with it. In one particularly touching example, I talked to the son of a resident who told me how a nursing home's social worker had prepared his mother for the arrival of his father, who was being transferred to the home from another facility. The preparations included taking her to the home's beauty shop the day before, helping her into her favorite clothes on the day of his arrival, and arranging for a welcoming committee and party. The son told me this story with tears welling in his eyes. Obviously, he was grateful for a staff that understood the emotional needs of people at such an important time in their lives.

The last set of questions is similar to those addressed to the other interviewees. Specifically, you need to learn why any deficiencies occurred and what was done to remedy them. Finally, there are the questions about strengths and weaknesses.

SOCIAL-SERVICES DIRECTOR QUESTIONNAIRE—
PRELIMINARY VISIT

I. Director's Education and Experience

    a. How long have you been director of social services? Are you full time or part-time in this position?

    b. What other social-services positions have you held?

    c. What is your educational background?

II. Social-Service Department Issues

    a. How many social workers or social-work assistants are employed in the department?

    b. What type of counseling services do you provide to the residents?

    c. What types of services do you provide to the families of residents?

    d. What are the typical problems new residents encounter when they first move into the home and what type of assistance does the home provide to deal with those problems?

III. The Home in General

    a. On the 19____ Medicare/Medicaid survey report, the following deficiencies were noted in social services: Could you please explain what happened to cause these deficiencies and how they were corrected?

    b. What do you see as the strengths of the home?

    c. What do you see as the weaknesses of the home?

❧

Interviewing the Activities Director

The quality of life in a nursing home will to a great extent be affected by the quality of a home's activities department. A trained activities director will probably have well-planned and executed programs. Vibrant, interesting, comprehensive, accessible, and available activity programs will do much to improve life for the residents. However, none of this can take place without staff and frequently also an active volunteer program.

The first two questions are designed to ascertain the commitment of resources that the nursing home is making to an activities program. The next three questions ask for specifics about the programs. Almost every nursing home issues a monthly schedule of activities—obtain the schedule and study it. Note how many different kinds of activities are offered at the home. Of these activities, how many are active and how many are passive? How many involve the residents truly interacting with other residents and staff and how many allow the residents simply to be observers? Are there special events that tie together weeks or months? Are there projects such as workshops or theater productions that allow the residents to build self-esteem while enjoying themselves? Finally, does everything end at 2:30 P.M., leaving the residents to fend for themselves in front of a television for the rest of the day?

To a great extent, the activities staff should be part of the total therapeutic team, and question (f) provides an opening to explore how the activities program fits into the rest of the nursing-home environment. Question (g) is similar to one asked in the social-services interview about new residents' adjustment problems. Here again, it would be useful to know what to expect and how insightful and resourceful the staff is at identifying and working out the inevitable adjustment problems.

The last section of this questionnaire includes the standard Medicare/Medicaid deficiency question, along with the strengths-and-weaknesses questions.

*   *   *

At the end of these staff interviews, you and your visiting team should have gleaned a range of answers that should be helpful in your decision-making about a nursing home.

ACTIVITIES DIRECTOR QUESTIONNAIRE—
PRELIMINARY VISIT

I. <u>Activities Department Issues</u>

    a. How many full-time staffers are assigned to the activities department?

    b. How many volunteers work in the activities area?

    c. What is the range of activities programs at the home?

    d. What are the programs during a typical month?

    e. What programs occur on weekends and evenings?

    f. What is the relationship between the activities department and physical therapy, occupational therapy, and social services?

    g. What are the typical problems new residents have in adjusting to the activities programs? What is done in the department to help them deal with these problems?

II. <u>The Home in General</u>

    a. On the 19____ Medicaid/Medicaire survey report, the following deficiencies were noted in activities: Could you please explain what happened to cause these deficiencies and how they were corrected?

    b. What do you see as the strengths of the home?

    c. What do you see as the weaknesses of the home?

Interviewing Some Residents

Nothing will prove to be more rewarding than interviewing nursing-home residents. Over the course of my travels, I have interviewed hundreds of residents, and with few exceptions, I have found them to be both insightful and articulate. The questions on the accompanying form are the types I have asked numerous times—ones that get to the heart of the matter about nursing homes. Although skeptics may suggest that any resident who is interested in speaking with visitors or whom an administration is willing to volunteer for an interview is going to be a proponent of the home, be prepared for some big surprises during interviews with residents. I have frequently found that after a few minutes of conversation, residents will open up and be quite candid about their nursing-home experiences. Indeed, I have become uncomfortable at times upon hearing of parents abandoned by their children and facilities where staff are unresponsive and constantly angling for tips. This information is essential to the decision-making process, and residents are particularly qualified to discuss the subject of life in the nursing home. The last question frequently is the most revealing. While some residents may be reluctant to criticize, almost all are willing to suggest what needs to be done to improve life at the home.

RESIDENT QUESTIONNAIRE—PRELIMINARY VISIT

I. Background Information

   a. How long have you lived at this home?

   b. Why did you move into this nursing home?

II. Resident Issues

   a. What do you like about the home?

   b. What do you dislike about the home?

   c. How is the food?

   d. Are the nurses responsive to your needs?

   e. Does the staff try to help you when necessary?

   f. Is the activities program interesting and stimulating?

   g. Are you satisfied with the housekeeping here?

   h. How would you characterize the other residents of the nursing home? Are they nice? Friendly? Kind? Considerate? Boring? Nasty? Withdrawn? Argumentative?

   i. What do the residents do to help new residents adjust to life in the nursing home?

   j. What were your problems in making the transition to life in the home?

   k. If you could change two things here, what would they be?

OBSERVATION DURING THE VISIT

On this first visit and tour, it is impossible to do and see everything. However, during the course of the visit, it is imperative that the team make some careful observations about the environment of the home, the condition of the residents, and the behavior of the staff vis-à-vis the residents. In the next several sections, I shall describe areas to address during the tour.

The Smell Test

Nursing homes should not smell of urine. If they do, a red flag should go up, because that means the home is not active enough in dealing with continence problems. When there are odor problems, it frequently means also that the home is understaffed in nursing or housekeeping and the smell has permeated the drapes, rugs, and sometimes the furniture. While the olfactory senses may fatigue after a while, the reality of staffing problems does not go away. So if a home fails the smell test, the problem may be serious. Finally, do not be deceived by floral fragrances introduced into the air circulation systems; they merely mask the stench of urine and the true situation of the home.

Cleanliness

During the tour and the visits to patients' rooms, observe how well housekeeping is taking care of the public hallways and the patient-care areas. Questions to be answered: Are bathrooms clean? Are floors and walls clean?

A good acid test is to check the dining room an hour or so after a meal. Has it been cleaned up? Is the floor free of food? Look carefully at the tables to see whether there is any food encrustation.

If there are housekeeping problems, note them and ask the administrator why they exist.

Observe the Residents

During the course of your visit, you will have numerous opportunities to observe residents. Begin by looking at their clothes. Are the residents dressed properly for the weather? Are their clothes neat, clean, and in good repair? Are residents properly dressed for the time of day? Is their hair well combed? Does it appear clean?

When you shake hands with a resident, observe the state of his or her fingernails. Are they clean and of a reasonable length? Look at the person's eyes. Are they free of crusts?

Look for signs of restraints, such as cloth straps on the beds and on wheelchairs. If you see a number of these, ask the nursing director about the home's policy on restraints.

Observe the Staff

As you tour the facility, observe the activity of the staff, particularly in the nursing unit. Are the nurses and aides working with the residents or are they busy at the nursing station writing in charts? What appears to be the relationship between the nurses and the residents? In some homes that I have visited, there is a clear sense of mutual respect and camaraderie between these two groups. In others, unfortunately, the staff acts as jailers and the residents behave like prisoners. A nursing home *must* be a place of dignity for the elderly, and the role of the staff is to serve the needs of the elderly in an efficient and effective manner. As you look around, try to collect evidence that can demonstrate how well the staff is doing its job at the home.

ANALYZING THE INFORMATION

Although the process outlined can be exhausting, it is absolutely the best way to gather the data necessary to make a reasoned decision. There are no shortcuts. The next step is analysis of the material.

Threshold Question

The first question that must be answered by all who are part of this decision is: Based on what you have observed, are you comfortable with the reality of a nursing home for the prospective resident? Are there alternatives other than nursing homes that should be explored? A related question may be: Are there other nursing homes that should receive a preliminary visit?

Tearing and Comparing

Finally it is time for all members of the team to compare notes about all the homes visited. It is best to prepare a simple summary chart that lists the strengths and weaknesses of the various homes visited and reaches some conclusions about the apparent quality of care and quality of life offered to residents at each home. This chart can be used as the basis for the family discussion about the best solution. Obviously, nothing should be held back in this discussion, which should result in the selection of one or more homes for a second round of visits.

The process I have outlined is likely to end with the elimination of one or more homes, so that perhaps one or more choices remain. Assuming agreement can be reached on one or two choices, then it's time to prepare for the second round.

No final decision should be made until after the second visit—the subject of the next chapter.

THE CRUCIAL
SECOND LOOK

If you only follow one of the many recommendations in this book, select this one: **Make a second visit to any nursing home that is being seriously considered!**

The goals of the second visit are to validate initial impressions, clarify the Medicare/Medicaid deficiency status of the nursing home, follow up on issues that may have come to mind after the first visit, and clarify the nature of any arrangements that need to be made prior to admission.

The reason the second visit turns out to be so important is simple: There is relatively little anxiety with the second trip because the people and the places are familiar. Nonetheless, as with the first set of interviews, the key to a successful visit is preparation. In this chapter, I discuss the strategy for being prepared and then suggest further issues to raise with various staff members and residents of the home.

BEING PREPARED:
Checking Out the Full Survey

The first step in being prepared for the second visit is to obtain the home's most recent Medicare/Medicaid survey report and the plan for correction of deficiencies. Despite the fact that these reports are public documents to which everyone theoretically has access, obtaining your own copy may require some tenacity. In some states, such as California and Oregon, the most recent report is required to be posted on a consumer information bulletin board near the entrance of the nursing home. In some homes that I visited in California, the form was indeed available and a visitor could easily pull it out of a pouch and read it—although photocopying might be more problematic. In other homes, the letter of the California law was met—that is, the report was on the board, but only the cover letter was showing, and the rest of the report was well secured with thumbtacks behind the cover letter (which itself was covered in plastic and secured on the bulletin board!). It would take a very determined person to stand at the board and dislodge that report. A second alternative is to ask the administrator of the home for a copy of the report. I tried that at several homes and received all kinds of evasive answers about its availability.

Probably the best way to get the report—if the home will not release a copy to you—is to contact the state agency responsible for conducting the Medicare/Medicaid survey. (A list and phone numbers are provided in Appendix 1.) Be forewarned, however—this route requires a bit of persistence. For example, in test runs in several states, it took me a number of calls and conversations to obtain the surveys and plans of corrections.

Once you have the surveys and the plans of corrections, review the plans and note the major problem areas. These problem areas should be organized so that you can discuss them with the administrator or other staff members when you make your second visit.

Recommendations from Residents and Families

The next step in the process is to obtain references about the nursing home from people who have experienced its services. There are two problems connected with this: First, you need to get the names of people who have had dealings with the home; this may be simple or it may require some ingenuity. It is simple when the home and you are part of the same community and you or members of your family or friends know current or former residents. However, the problem of obtaining names is more complex when you are a stranger, although several options exist. Start with the home's social workers, and ask them whether they can provide the names of people who are involved with the home's activities and could serve as references. If that doesn't work, ask members of the local clergy if they know of any people in the community whom you could call for references. Another option is to call the local hospital and ask its social worker or discharge planner for names of potential reference givers. The hospital staff might also be able to provide the names of physicians who have patients at the home. Finally, if all else fails, contact the residents you met on the preliminary visit and ask them for names of several people whom you can call.

Once you have established your calling list, it is best to speak (either face to face or on the phone) with each person and gather the information suggested on the basic Reference Form—Residents and Families, which accompanies this chapter. This form merely identifies the person who is giving the reference and suggests several questions geared toward opening the discussion about the home. Next, there are specific questions about nursing, therapies, activities, administration, social services, food, and environment/sanitation. Each of these questions is designed to probe the experiences of the reference provider. It helps to ask the provider to identify specific examples, because by asking for these in addition to conclusions, you are in a better position to evaluate the weight you wish to assign to the reference. Finally, ask the reference giver if it is acceptable to call again if other questions come to mind. In some cases, another member of the decision group or perhaps the potential resident may wish to make the follow-up call.

REFERENCE FORM—RESIDENTS AND FAMILIES

Date _____

Reference's Name _____ Phone # _____

QUESTIONS

1. What is the nature of your contact with the nursing home?
2. Why did you (or your family) select this home?
3. Did you consider other homes in the area? Which ones? Why were they rejected?
4. How long have you [or your family member] resided in the home?
5. What type of care are you receiving (skilled, intermediate, or custodial)?
6. What has been your experience with the home?
7. Could you provide specific examples of positive and negative experiences you have had with the care at the home?
8. Is the nursing staff competent? Responsive?
9. Do you feel that the activities program is sufficiently interesting and stimulating? Can you provide examples?
10. Has the therapy program (physical therapy, occupational therapy, art therapy, music therapy) proved to be interesting, stimulating, and/or helpful? Can you provide examples?
11. Is the administration responsive when you have problems? Can you provide examples?
12. Has the social-services department been helpful or not? Can you provide specific examples?
13. How is the food at the nursing home?
14. How is the general environment of the place? Is it clean and free of odors? Is it homelike or institutional? Is it a cheerful place?

CLOSING QUESTION

15. May I or a member of my family call you again if we have some additional questions?

Reference Taker _____

Recommendations from Care Providers

Present and even former providers of care at the nursing home can be an invaluable source of information about what goes on at the facility. There are two problems likely to be encountered in securing these recommendations. First, it frequently is difficult to identify the caregivers unless you are in a small community. Second, once you have identified some potential reference givers, it often is difficult to elicit candid opinions. In this section are some suggestions about dealing with these problems, and the Reference Form—Caregivers (at the end of this section) offers some questions that may overcome the natural reticence of these people to discuss their present or former organization.

Handling the first of these problems—that is, identifying knowledgeable caregivers—is primarily a matter of persistence. By doggedly calling a number of people, you undoubtedly will be able to identify several physicians, nurses, and therapists who have worked closely with the nursing home. Several starting points might be a family physician or friends who work in the local hospital as social workers, nurses, or therapists. Even if you do not know anyone in the community, you could stop by or call the local hospital and ask people in the social-services department for suggestions. Another contact is the local Council on the Elderly (or whatever name it uses). Stop by their offices and ask the staff to help you identify potential sources of references. If you are living in a large city, local clergy may be helpful, as will politicians, who make their living by knowing what is happening in their communities. In smaller towns, selectmen and other officials may be able to point you in the proper direction.

When you have identified several potential contacts, the next challenge is to get in touch with them and establish enough rapport so they will provide you with the answers you are seeking. Again, making contact is a matter of persistence. Begin by calling at the person's office, and if you cannot connect at the time, leave a message and a phone number. If you are out of town, place a person-to-person call and advise the other party to call back collect. If you do not have a response within a day or two, make a second call—and a third one if necessary. Consider telephoning early in the morning (before eight) or later in the afternoon (after five)—often those are the best times to catch busy people. If all else fails, and the reference promises to be a crucial one, consider calling the person at home in the evening. While most of us do not wish to be disturbed then, remember that the stakes in this situation are very high and the decision you make has profound implications for everyone.

Once you have made contact, I suggest you spend a minute outlining your situation so that the person can have a frame of reference for his or her response. On the Reference Form— Caregivers is an outline of information you might want to provide prior to the questions. Next, a series of semi–open-ended questions may help the caregiver to focus his or her experiences in the nursing home as well as his or her analysis of the quality of care and quality of life at the home. Then I suggest you ask two closing questions, both of which request the reference provider to stand in your shoes and make a judgment about the home in terms of your needs. Obviously, the person at the other end of the phone does not have the total information about the potential resident but these two questions do provide an opportunity for him or her to think about the home and your situation in a concrete manner. A response to the last question which suggests other homes may be particularly significant. For example, it would not be surprising if a present or former staff member would in his or her reluctance to talk to a stranger about the home give out a mixed message of praise for the home but a suggestion that you look at other places. Such a suggestion should be viewed as an indicator that the home has problems that should be investigated.

REFERENCE FORM—CAREGIVERS

Date _____

Reference's Name _____ Phone # _____

I. *Rapport Building* [It is suggested that you begin the conversation by describing the condition of the potential resident.]

Suggested opening "Dr./Mr./Ms. _____ , I am sorry to bother you but I have a problem that you may be able to help me with (and your name was suggested to me by _____) because of your association and experience with the _____ nursing home.

Condition of potential resident

a. My family is presently looking for a nursing home for my mother, who is _____ years old

b. She needs (total/some/no) assistance with the following activities of daily living:
   eating
   bathing
   toileting
   transferring
   dressing

c. Her medical diagnosis is:

QUESTIONS

1. What type of involvement have you had with the _____ nursing home?

2. What is your impression of the quality of care provided at the home?

3. Can you provide examples of good or poor care given at the home?

4. What is your impression of the quality of life at the home for residents? Can you provide examples of good or poor aspects?

CLOSING QUESTIONS

5. From what I have told you about my mother, do you think the _____ nursing home would be a good placement?

6. Could you suggest any other nursing homes in the area that would be a better place for my mother?

Reference Taker _____

❧

USING THE DATA FROM THE REFERENCES

The data from the references will be all negative, all positive, or mixed. Consistently negative reviews should cause you to contemplate eliminating this home from your list. If competent, experienced witnesses all have found the home wanting, there is a high probability that you would also be dissatisfied with it. While it is possible that the reference givers are biased and do not see the strengths of the home, or perhaps they have a vendetta against the home, the more likely explanation is that the home is of poor quality. Although it is difficult to go back to square one, it probably is a wiser course of action than settling for an inadequate facility and the hassles that you will encounter in trying to make such a home responsive to your needs.

Reviews that are all positive or mixed provide guidance for the second site visit. In both instances, the primary value of the reference check will be to identify areas for further inquiry on your second visit. For example, if several people point up problems with a boring and pedestrian activities program, you may want to spend extra time looking into that. On the other hand, if everyone raves about the food, it probably is not worth making an effort to examine the food services at the home.

Regardless of the findings, this second visit is absolutely necessary. The next section covers that visit, proposing what areas need exploration and including a list of suggested questions.

THE SECOND VISIT

The second visit to a nursing home will likely be more useful than the first one. The anxiety will be significantly diminished because you will be familiar with the home and its people. Also, you will be a more experienced and sophisticated visitor than on your first visit. But, just as with the first visit, it will be necessary to call the administrator (or in some cases the admitting office) to arrange the interviews and tour.

Old Places: Dozens of New Questions

This second visit provides the opportunity to probe areas of concern and clarify ambiguities about care at the home. From the survey documents that you have read, some questions should already be in mind (better yet, written down). In addition, you should consider asking the questions that appear on the accompanying Second-Visit Questionnaire. Most of these are the same or similar to questions that trained interviewers ask when they visit the nursing home. In many instances, the proper answers are obvious, and in all instances, the answers will clarify how the nursing home is treating residents and how it is likely to treat a new resident.

SECOND-VISIT QUESTIONNAIRE

A. Questions for Residents

1. How long have you lived in this nursing home? Why are you here?

2. What responsibilities do you have in living here? How were you informed about these responsibilities?

3. If there are changes in services or costs, does someone explain these?

4. To what extent has your doctor talked to you about your health and your treatment?

5. Do you know that you can refuse treatment or medication?

6. Have you or has anyone you know at the nursing home ever refused treatment or medication? If yes, what happened to you or to them?

7. Are the staff and administration responsive to complaints? To whom can you complain?

8. Does the nursing home hold any money that belongs to you? How easy or difficult is it for you to obtain that money?

9. Has anything been stolen from you while at the nursing home? What did the staff or administration do about it?

10. Have you ever been restrained? If yes, why were you restrained? Do you know why you were restrained?

11. Do you feel safe in this facility?

12. What degree of privacy and respect do you receive?

13. Can you have visits and phone calls from anyone? Is there adequate privacy in the nursing home?

14. What are your favorite activities at the home?

15. Is participation optional or required?

16. Do you have any trouble getting to off-campus activities?

17. Do you know of any resident who was transferred out of the home? Why was he/she transferred? To your knowledge, was the transfer discussed with the resident and his/her family before the move?

18. How often does your personal physician visit? Is it often enough? If you want to see your doctor, is it easily arranged?

19. If you have bowel or bladder problems, what type of help do you get from the staff?

20. If you need help getting to the toilet, how long do you need to wait to be taken there?

21. Do residents generally feel that people taking care of them know what they are doing? If no, please explain.

22. How long do you usually wait for help when you put your call light on?

23. What assistance do you need in the following areas, and if you do need assistance, who provides it? Bathing, dressing, eating, getting into and out of bed, getting in and out of a wheelchair, going to the toilet.

24. Do you feel that the assistance provided to you is done in an appropriate manner? For example, if you need help getting into or out of bed, do you feel safe when being helped?

25. If you have trouble sleeping, can you get assistance? What type of assistance?

26. Is you cane, crutch, or walker comfortable for you to use?

27. Do you always receive your medications on time? Does the nurse stay with you as you take your medications?

28. How is the food? Is it tasty? Are the portions sufficient? How do you get food outside of regular meal times?

29. How often does someone from dietary visit you to ask about your opinions on the food service?

30. Do you receive any kind of therapy here, such as physical therapy, occupational therapy, or speech therapy? If yes, why do you receive the therapy? How long have you received the therapy? Where do you receive the therapy? What happens if the therapist is absent?

31. Is your room kept clean? What about the rest of the nursing home?

32. If you could make some changes around the nursing home, what would they be?

B. Questions for Nurses

1. What is the standard procedure if a resident claims that something was stolen from him or her?

2. How do you get medical information and orders on a new resident?

3. How often do physicians normally visit residents in the home?

4. Who are the physicians with the most residents in the home? How much time do they spend with a resident on a typical visit?

5. How do you choose what clothing each of your residents wears each day? What do you do if a resident insists on wearing dirty or mismatched clothes?

6. What is the schedule for bathing residents and washing hair?

7. Does the nursing home have a special bowel and bladder training program?

8. Do you think that there is enough help in this nursing home? If no, why not?

9. What do you do about residents who are having trouble sleeping?

10. How many residents receive physical therapy, occupational therapy, or speech therapy?

C. Questions for Administration

1. How do residents learn what is expected of them?

2. How do residents learn of changes in the nursing home's procedures or charges?

3. Is the nursing home participating in any research projects that directly or indirectly involve residents? If yes, what are these projects? How many residents are involved? What arrangements are made to secure their informed consent?

4. What is the facility's policy concerning restraints? Do you make a distinction between safety devices and restraints? If so, what is the policy for safety devices?

5. Who trains staff in use of restraints?

6. What type of activities go on during the evening hours and on weekends?

7. Who is notified if a resident is injured?

8. What is the nursing home's policy on notifying a relative or responsible other party if a resident's condition changes?

9. What is the nursing home's policy regarding physician visits?

10. Have any physicians on your medical staff been disciplined? If yes, why?

11. Who provides therapy to the home's residents?

12. How many people were transferred out of this nursing home to another nursing home within the past year? What were the circumstances of the transfer?

D. Questions for Social-Services Staff

1. How are roommate assignments made? What is the process for changing roommates or room assignments? To what extent does cost enter into the decision about room assignment?

2. What is done to maintain resident dignity?

3. How is transportation arranged for off-campus activities?

4. Do residents participate in their plans for care?

5. How often does social services meet with a resident's family?

6. How often does social services meet with nursing?

7. How frequently do residents get out of the facility for activities?

Areas for Observation

During the course of this second visit, it is imperative to observe carefully what is happening at the nursing home. Here are areas for particular attention:

1. Do you see any examples of obviously inappropriate roommate situations, such as an alert resident rooming with a noisy and confused person?

2. Are the interactions between the staff and residents free of harassment, threats, and humiliation?

3. Are there areas for residents to be alone or meet in private with friends and relatives?

4. Are residents appropriately dressed for the time of day and the weather?

5. Do resident rooms appear to be deinstitutionalized with some personal furniture or other belongings?

6. Is there enough space to store clothing?

7. Are residents clean and free of odors? Is there crusting around their eyelids? Are eyeglasses properly fitted and clean? Are there dried food particles or drool around the mouth? Does hair appear to be clean and combed or brushed? Are nails clean and of the appropriate length?

8. If you see a resident in need of assistance, is that resident being assisted? Is it being done in a safe and competent manner? Does the staff appear to be minimizing pain and discomfort while assisting the resident?

9. Does the facility have grab bars in all the corridors?

10. Are the resident rooms functional? Do the bathrooms have grab bars around the toilets?

11. Observe—better yet, eat a meal in—the residents' dining hall. Observe whether there is enough time for the meal. Is assistance provided to those people who need it? Are any adaptive eating devices being used? Are resident's clothes being protected? Is there adequate space in the dining room and at the table?

12. Ask to see sample menus that cover a week or more. Check for variety.

13. Ask for a tour of the kitchen. Look for rust on shelves, dripping or spillage on shelves or floors, or dirty food-preparation equipment.

14. Ask for a tour of the therapy area. Does the equipment appear to be clean and in good working order?

15. Finally, observe the general condition of the home. Is the paint chipped? Are the public spaces clean and free of odors? Are the bathrooms in good repair?

DECISIONS AND DEALS

Now comes the hardest part of the process—making a decision and finalizing the deal. The decision amounts to this: After comparing several nursing homes, which one will provide the best quality of care and quality of life for the resident? The data collected from the various references and the two visits will most often point in one direction. By conducting the type of in-depth research and analysis suggested in this book, family members will be able to distance themselves from the superficial considerations that frequently cause people to choose a facility that looks good initially but turns out later to be problematic. You can avoid this if you are a prudent buyer and make your decision on the basis of substance, not superficial amenities.

Once the selection is made, it is absolutely imperative to obtain a copy of the contract that you will be expected to sign with the nursing home. **Do Not Sign This Contract Without Carefully Reviewing And, If Appropriate, Questioning Each Word And Sentence In It.** You may want to hire an attorney to read the contract and negotiate any changes—the time to make changes is *before* admission. After admission, there is practically no leverage for making a contract change.

In Appendix 2 are copies of several admission agreements, including the one required under California law. This document, while long enough to give most people (lawyers included) a headache, is worth reading because it provides a useful model. It is particularly excellent in the area of incidental and extra expenses, which often can run in excess of $1000 per month.

If you have a major medical problem, going to the Mayo Clinic in Rochester, Minnesota, may make a great deal of sense. But if you need a nursing home, you do not have to go to a medical mecca, since there may be an excellent facility in your community or only a short ride away. In the next chapter, I will focus on the elements of an excellent nursing home and share my experiences of visiting some of the nation's best facilities.

TEN

FINDING A FIRST-CLASS NURSING HOME:
The Elements of Excellence

INTRODUCTION

This book began as an inquiry into those elements that make a nursing home an outstanding place as well as a search for the "best" nursing home in America. I thought that if I could find, analyze, and describe the "best," it could become the model for the nation's other homes.

I was wrong! Despite my expectations, I did not find the one "best" home in America. Instead, I encountered numerous excellent homes—places I would recommend without reservation. These homes were in dozens of communities from Portland, Oregon, to Portland, Maine, southern California to southern Florida, and myriad points in between. Indeed, I doubt that there even is a best home; rather, what exists are many homes with excellent and unusual programs and staffs, but no one home has it all. This chapter summarizes the essence of this book by identifying nine elements of an excellent nursing home and presenting some supporting examples.

ELEMENT 1: Mission

It is absolutely obvious to me that first-class nursing homes are those where there is a clear mission related to some philosophical, religious, or patriotic commitment. Whether it is the government-owned nursing home at the Audie Murphy Memorial Veterans Hospital in San Antonio or the Advent Christian Church's religiously oriented nursing home in Vernon,

Vermont, what I have seen at these and many other excellent homes is a special focus on mission.

Sometimes that focus is manifested in a well-articulated philosophy, such as the one Dr. Herbert Shore developed at Golden Acres in Dallas, that is displayed prominently in the home's lobby as a constant reminder to residents, staff, family, and visitors:

> Care at Golden Acres is expressed by *L*ove, *I*nterest, *F*ulfillment, and *E*nrichment. This L.I.F.E. philosophy forms the foundation of services you, as the resident, receive. The basic objective of our program is *to add life to years, not just years to life.*
>
> At Golden Acres we feel that aging is a normal process that need not be a period of physical and mental deterioration. As an individual, you will be treated with dignity and understanding. We believe that to care *for* you, we must care *about* you and understand that you are deserving of courtesy and respect. We hope that you will feel that the attitude of the staff is one of dedication to maintaining your optimal level of functioning. In this endeavor, the Golden Acres staff seeks to plan with you and your family, a rehabilitation-resocialization program that emphasizes your abilities and not disabilities.

At other homes, the focus is maintained through the simple act of prayer. Kent Kirkwood is the director of Resthaven, a 271-bed nursing home in Independence, Missouri, owned by the Reorganized Church of Jesus Christ of Latter Day Saints. He begins his morning management meetings with a short prayer to focus the meeting on the true meaning of the home, which he views as "ministering to the people."

Perhaps the best philosophy is the one that no one should be in a nursing home unless it is absolutely necessary. It is also one that is not attempting to "sell" the nursing home but rather to assist people in the search for programmatic alternatives to nursing-home care. In Beechwood, Ohio, I talked to Harvey Shankman, director of social services at Menorah Park Nursing Home, who said, "We're here to help." What this means in practice is that an interview with Shankman or a member of his staff begins with an exploration of alternatives, such as day-care programs, respite centers, home care, congregate housing, or home-delivered meals.

Sometimes the commitment comes out in less noticeable ways. For example, I attended the meeting of the board of directors' executive committee of a not-for-profit nursing home where the subject was recruitment of an activities staff person for the Alzheimer's unit. The recommendation presented to the committee was to hire a part-time activities person for the unit. This was challenged by one member, who argued that, despite the home's projected $250,000 deficit, it was in the best interests of the unit's residents to have a full-time activities person. Finally, he noted, "So we are $250,000 in the hole; we'll be another $12,000 deeper." His recommendation was accepted.

ELEMENT 2: Economic Orientation

While this is a country committed to free-enterprise capitalism, and the profit motive may give us better disposable diapers or department stores, it does not work so well in the area of long-term care for the elderly.

To put it bluntly, you are more likely to get the most substantive value for your nursing-home dollars in a government-owned facility or a not-for-profit home owned by an organization rooted in a religious or charitable trust. As noted in chapter 1, government and not-for-profit homes, which are not attempting to earn an income for investors, inevitably have higher staffing ratios, active volunteer programs (which add staff without cost), and frequently operate at a deficit, which is covered through active fund-raising programs or income from endowments. One of the best bargains in nursing homes is the Veterans Administration, which operates cheerful and well-staffed places such as the Audie Murphy Home in San Antonio and other homes located throughout the country. Local chapters of the Masons and the Odd Fellows also own excellent homes. For example, I visited a fine Odd Fellows home in Portland, Oregon, that had a residential-care facility attached to it; in Wallingford, Connecticut, I visited the Masonic Home, part of a large complex that includes retirement apartments and a hospital. Despite the complex's size, the Masonic Home is an integral part of this total community. The home's residents derive many advantages from being on such a campus with its myriad programs and high staffing ratio, particularly in the clinical areas.

An unfortunate reality is that in many parts of the country, Medicaid does not allow a nursing home to be profitable unless the home cuts corners and provides staff exactly at state minimum levels. In many states, residents of homes that cater to Medicaid beneficiaries will have limited services, and both the quality-of-life activities and the quality of care will be barely adequate, at best.

Since money appears to be a crucial factor in whether or not one can get into a nursing home, it is frequently difficult to have the option of choosing between "sizzle" and "steak" in nursing homes. Careful applicants sometimes can get both. The trick is simple—do not be hoodwinked by plush lobbies, grand pianos, and reproduction antique furniture. These facilities frequently are targeting their marketing to guilt-ridden children—"Mom, look at this beautiful hotel you will be in. . . ." On the other hand, the well-staffed, well-organized place may choose to make its investment in staff and programs, not in assuaging the children's guilt.

ELEMENT 3: Governance

An active governing board makes a big difference. While the not-for-profits and many government homes have boards, there is nothing to preclude a privately owned nursing home from establishing, at a minimum, an advisory board. Such boards, governing or advisory, meet periodically to monitor and evaluate the functioning of the institution. A good board that is knowledgeable and concerned about the nursing home and does not have a personal financial stake in the facility brings a measure of oversight and ideas that can be very useful.

In Portland, Oregon, I met with the board leadership of the Robison Home, one of the best smaller facilities that I visited on my various trips. Typical of other high-quality and concerned boards was their question: How did I think that their home could be improved? I have always found that the best homes are interested both in constructive criticism and in getting even better. A statement that is typical of board members' attitudes was recently published in *WATCH*, the newsletter of San Antonio's Morningside Ministries. One of the members summarized her feelings about the board by stating, "The individual members come to meetings with a religious commitment to providing the very best in quality care for older people."

In sum, the practice of interested outsiders regularly looking over management's shoulder appears to be directly connected to excellence.

ELEMENT 4: A Real Medical Staff

In chapter 1, I outlined the various options that homes have for staffing their facilities. Since residents normally have the freedom to select their own personal physician, the issue is what the nursing home does to ensure that the performance of the attending physicians is adequate and that the overall quality of care in the home is appropriate to the needs of the residents. In light of the increasing needs of the elderly, all but the smallest nursing homes certainly need more than a token presence of a medical director.

In practice, this means that a home with more than a hundred beds probably needs a quarter- to a half-time medical director—that is, someone in the home ten to twenty hours per week dealing with the issues of quality of care, recertification, staff training, drug therapy, bowel and bladder problems, patient care, and family concerns. The prevalent system of hit-and-miss medical care is simply unconscionable.

ELEMENT 5: Adequate Nursing

Nurses are the heart of a nursing home. All of the excellent homes I saw had staffing ratios that exceeded state minimums—some by as much as 40 percent. In Acadia, California, I visited the Huntington Avenue Convalescent Hospital, a facility owned by Beverly Enterprises. At this small but pleasant nursing home across the road from the Santa Anita racetrack, there were 3.5 nursing hours per resident per day—considerably above the California requirements. While many other homes also exceeded these requirements, only one, the Audie Murphy Home in San Antonio, was staffed entirely by licensed nurses—rather unusual and extremely expensive. But, as Beverly Enterprises demonstrates, even profit-oriented nursing homes can deliver care in decent physical surroundings with adequate staffing ratios.

With regard to nurses, there are several concerns. First, does the home have enough? Ratios in excess of 3.0 hours per day per resident, based on my experience, have been acceptable. The second question is: Does the home have the appropriate mix of staff? The first-class homes have experienced registered nurses, or at least licensed nurses, on duty around the clock. Related to this is the question of the depth that a home has. For example, is more than one licensed person on duty each night? The point is simple: The licensed nurses have the training and maturity to deal with almost all of the problems likely to come up during a given day. The aides simply do not have the training or the experience to deal with many problems that could mean the difference between living and dying or pehaps between a night of comfort and a night of agony.

The final issue is whether the home has recruited people with the appropriate level of experience and maturity to handle the jobs. For example, at one privately owned home in Texas, I met the evening supervisor, an RN who held a master's degree and also was a recently retired colonel from the nurse corps of the U.S. Army. Knowing that such an experienced and qualified person is on duty in the evening builds confidence in an institution. All of the excellent homes were filled with people who were interested and committed to the elderly and who frequently had advanced training in a range of gerontological specialties.

ELEMENT 6: Therapeutic Services

Many nursing homes either provide or arrange for the basic physical- and occupational-therapy services described in chapter 1. Excellence exists when a home provides these services with full-time therapists and aides, and also when these services are easily accessible to the residents—that is, they are essentially part of the institution's routine program. Frankly, many homes only provide the therapeutic services on a contract basis if there is an additional private or Medicare payment for the services. Unfortunately, when this is the case, those who cannot afford the services will experience a slow but steady loss of strength and functioning as a result.

An excellent home also provides a broad range of additional therapeutic services that deal with the physical and emotional needs of the residents. Among these are social-service counseling for residents and their families, art therapy, gardening therapy, pet therapy, music therapy, and dance therapy. It should be reemphasized that there is a world of difference between the activities of art therapy and the typical painting activity prevalent in many homes. Painting or sculpting may be good "therapy," but at Kansas City's Shalom Geriatric Center and a number of other places, it is part of a program to diagnose and treat a range of emotional programs. The therapists at Shalom and elsewhere are part of the clinical-care team whose observations and analyses are used by social workers, nurses, and physicians to develop and modify treatment plans.

In addition to having the right staff, a good therapy program needs facilities and equipment. A physical-therapy or occupational-therapy program simply needs space that is comfortable, where therapists can work with residents. Even a well-organized garden-therapy program needs more than just a plot of earth. For example, at several homes there were raised garden boxes, which allowed residents to maneuver their wheelchairs close enough so they could reach in and do their work.

Overall, the therapeutic programs provide a bulwark against emotional and physical deterioration. The truly excellent homes *do* provide those services without a major concern about the costs.

ELEMENT 7: Activities

All nursing homes have bingo, a game I have come to detest. Indeed, bingo is the central activity in many homes. In speaking with nursing-home staff about the game, I have been told many times that it is what the residents want. In my judgment, it is not what is wanted but what is given.

Even the excellent homes have bingo. But they also have a great deal more—they have action. For example, in Kansas City, a home takes its residents on weekly trips to a local restaurant for pie and coffee. The Jewish Center for the Aged in St. Louis schedules more than 100 off-campus trips a year, including visits to shopping centers, the zoo, and concerts. Homes I visited in Connecticut and Cleveland sponsored camping trips to state parks for residents. One home takes residents to a resort hotel for a vacation from the nursing home. Friendship Village in Chesterfield, Missouri, runs intergenerational programs with the local schools, including a pen-pals club. Other homes have arrangements with local summer camps whereby teenage volunteers simply talk with the residents a few times a week. Several other homes operate sheltered workshops for residents where they can participate in a range of supervised projects and earn spending money. At Four Courts in Louisville, Kentucky, a local band has free rehearsal space each week, so it becomes a regular activity for the residents to watch and listen to the rehearsing musicians.

Among the best activities and programs I have seen are the following: At the Masonic Home in Wallingford, Connecticut, an extraordinary HO model train room has hundreds of cars and miles of track that residents can play with or work on; at Morningside Ministries in San Antonio, a lowered basketball hoop allows Alzheimer's residents to play outside without the usual frustration of shooting up to a ten-foot-high hoop; at the Riverview Home in Pittsburgh, there is an outdoor walking path and exercise course for residents; also in Pittsburgh, at the Forbes Geriatric Center, computers are available for residents to play games as well as to make personalized greeting cards; and the Robison Home in Portland, Oregon, has an indoor play area for visiting grandchildren and other youngsters. The list of creative and energetic programs I saw around the country is almost endless. The key to the excellent facility, though, is that it is interested in being a stimulating home for its residents, not merely a warehouse where the elderly wait to die.

ELEMENT 8: Physical Facilities

The best nursing homes I visited were always well maintained, bright, and cheerful. Some of them take a special interest in the art that is placed throughout the home. For example, at the Jewish Home in Worcester, Massachusetts, Marvin Goldberg, the director, has amassed an unusual and interesting collection that is displayed throughout the facility. In fact, it is worth a trip to Worcester to see his excellent nursing home as well as its superb collection of Andy Warhol prints.

Many homes have beauty parlors and barbershops, indoor and outdoor greenhouses, chapels, in-house cable-television systems, libraries, and snack bars and gift shops that sell a range of items from sugar-free candy to clothes.

In terms of design and total space, I was most impressed by such homes as Cleveland's Menorah Park, Seattle's Keiro, and Seattle's Kline Galland, which had many private sitting alcoves as well as large public spaces available for residents and their guests. Another well-designed facility in terms of public spaces is Miami's Douglas Gardens, where you enter a lobby with a snack bar directly ahead and a large and comfortable living room to the right. Because of the living room's size and design, it is possible for many family groups to sit and visit in relative privacy.

In terms of the residents' own rooms, I was always impressed with the homes that encouraged residents to create their own private spaces with pictures, a piece of furniture from home, or a favorite bedcover. Since many residents wind up sharing a room, it was particularly interesting to see the new quarters at the Jewish Home in Reseda, California, where beds in narrow, elongated rooms are essentially toe to toe so that each resident of a double room has access to a window.

ELEMENT 9: Top-Level Managerial Sensitivity

Perhaps what most distinguishes the truly excellent facility from the fair or poor home is the sensitivity of top management to the needs of the elderly and the translation of that sensitivity into action. The best example of this comes from an experience I had eighteen years ago in a small town in England, where I was visiting a 200-bed nursing home built on the edge of a new development. Within weeks of the home's opening, it filled to capacity, and the management experienced the problem of old men wandering away in the early evening hours. Eventually they were all located in the pubs in their old neighborhoods, and the home's solution is a case study in sensitivity, responsiveness, and creativity. The nursing home established its own pub, which was opened to the neighborhood. Soon the home became the focal point for neighborhood gatherings and the home's residents no longer had to be chased down throughout the town.

The band rehearsal space that Four Courts in Kentucky provides and the food and architecture of Seattle's Keiro Home are examples of sensitivity. Outdoor and indoor play space for children visiting grandparents (or, more likely, great-grandparents) is an indication of responsiveness to the needs of a family. Making it possible for family and friends to share special occasions—such as Easter, Christmas, or Passover—at the nursing home is another example.

Other managers make it their business to stay in touch with the residents by walking around the home several times a week and keeping in contact with the families. For example, at Morningside Ministries, Robert Freestate and his staff hold monthly family socials, which serve varying communication and support functions. As one way of interacting with his residents, Sheldon Blumenthal, director of the Jewish Home in Reseda, California, teaches classes for residents in current events and often leads religious services.

Many homes now have photos or collages of residents posted on their doors. Sometimes they contain biographical material, invaluable information for developing a sense of community and helping staff to understand the residents better. A number of homes have active videotaping programs in which family members can make tapes recollecting family events. These tapes can be shown to residents who become agitated— apparently a helpful technique for dealing with some forms of dementia.

Finally, the sensitive management is an advocate of residents rights (Appendix 3). For such management staff, these rights are not merely federal or state legal requirements but rather a code that ensures the dignity of life for the elderly.

A FINAL WORD

As I travel around the country, I frequently ask members of large groups how many of them expect to spend the last few years of their lives in a nursing home. Usually no one raises a hand. When a brave soul does say that he or she expects it to happen, it usually is because that person has a loved one in a good nursing home. A good—or, better yet, an excellent—home is not a place to fear, but rather a place to live. I will have done my job if this book helps you move closer to finding that excellent home.

RESOURCE NAMES, ADDRESSES, AND PHONE NUMBERS

NATIONAL AGENCIES AND ORGANIZATIONS

National Nursing-Home Organizations

American Association of Homes for the Aging
1129 20th Street, NW
Washington, DC 20036
(202) 296-5960

Note: This is the association of not-for-profit nursing homes.

American Health Care Association
1201 L Street, NW
Washington, DC 20005
(202) 842-4444

Note: This is the association of for-profit nursing homes.

National Resource Organizations

American Baptist Homes and Hospitals
Box 851
Valley Forge, PA 19482
(215) 768-2382

American Hospital Association
840 N. Lake Shore Drive
Chicago, IL 60611
(312) 280-6000

American Protestant Health Association
1701 E. Woodfield Road
Schaumburg, IL 60195
(312) 843-2701

Catholic Health Care Association of the United States
4455 Woodson Road
St. Louis, MO 63134
(314) 427-2500

Episcopal Society for Ministry on Aging
ESMA Sayre Hall
317 Wyandotte Street
Bethlehem, PA 18015
(215) 868-5400

Federation of Protestant Welfare Agencies
281 Park Avenue South
New York, NY 10010
(212) 777-4800

The Gerontological Society of America
1411 K Street, NW
Washington, DC 20005
(202) 393-1411

Lutheran Aging Services
810 E. Wisconsin Avenue
Deland, FL 32720
(904) 734-0601

Lutheran Hospitals and Homes Society
Box 2087
1202 Westrac Drive
Fargo, ND 58107
(701) 293-9053

National Association for Home Care
519 C Street, NW, Stanton Park
Washington, DC 20002
(202) 547-7424

North American Association of Jewish Homes and Housing for
the Aging
2525 Centerville Road
Dallas, TX 75228
(214) 328-0274

Federal Agencies

Division of Disability, Aging and Long Term Care
U.S. Department of Health and Human Services
200 Independence Avenue, SW
Washington, DC 20201
(202) 245-6172

Administration on Aging
U.S. Department of Health and Human Services
330 Independence Avenue, SW
Washington, DC 20201
(202) 245-0724

Health Care Financing Administration
Division of Medicare Eligibility Policy
U.S. Department of Health and Human Services
East High Rise Building
6325 Security Boulevard
Baltimore, MD 21207
(301) 966-4472

Health Care Financing Administration
Division of Medicaid Eligibility Policy
U.S. Department of Health and Human Services
East High Rise Building
6325 Security Boulevard
Baltimore, MD 21207
(301) 966-4452

Health Care Financing Administration
Division of Long Term Care Experiments
U.S. Department of Health and Human Services
Oak Meadows Building
6340 Security Boulevard
Baltimore, MD 21207
(301) 966-6649

National Institute on Aging
9000 Rockville Pike
Rockville, MD 20892
(301) 496-9265

Social Security Administration
6401 Security Boulevard
Baltimore, MD 21235
(301) 594-6660

Veterans Administration
Assistant Chief Medical Director for Geriatrics and Extended
Care
810 Vermont Avenue, NW
Washington, DC 20420
(202) 233-3781

STATE RESOURCES

Alabama

Health
Department of Public Health
434 Monroe Street
Montgomery, AL 36130
(205) 261-5052

Aging
Commission on Aging
Second Floor
136 Catoma Street
Montgomery, AL 36130
(205) 242-5743

Medicaid
Medicaid Agency
2500 Fairlane Drive
Montgomery, AL 36130
(205) 277-2710

Nonprofit Association
Alabama Association of Homes for the Aging
c/o Methodist Homes for the Aging
1424 Montclair Road
Birmingham, AL 35210
(205) 956-4150

Alaska

Health
Division of Public Health
P.O. Box H-06
Juneau, AK 99811
(907) 465-3090

Aging
Older Alaskans Commission
Department of Administration
Pouch C
Juneau, AK 99811
(907) 465-3250

Medicaid
Department of Health and Social Services
350 Main Street
P.O. Box H-01
Juneau, AK 99811
(907) 465-3030

Arizona

Health
Department of Health Services
1740 W. Adams Street
Phoenix, AZ 85007
(602) 542-1024

Aging
Aging and Adult Administration
Department of Economic Security
P.O. Box 6123
Phoenix, AZ 85005
(602) 542-4446

Medicaid
Arizona Health Care Cost Containment System
801 E. Jefferson
Phoenix, AZ 85034
(602) 234-3655

Nonprofit Associations
Arizona Association of Homes for the Aging
204 Abacus Tower
3030 North Third Street
Phoenix, AZ 85012
(602) 264-1984

Arkansas

Health
Arkansas Department of Health
4815 W. Markham Street
Little Rock, AR 72205-3867
(501) 661-2111

Aging
Office on Aging and Adult Services
Department of Human Services
Donaghey Building, 7th & Main Streets
Little Rock, AR 72201
(501) 682-2441

Medicaid
Department of Human Services
Division of Economic and Medical Services
7th & Main Streets, P.O. Box 1437
Little Rock, AR 72203
(501) 682-8650

California

Health
Department of Health Services
714 P Street
Sacramento, CA 95814
(916) 445-1248

Aging
Department on Aging
1020 19th Street
Sacramento, CA 95814
(916) 322-5290

Medicaid
Department of Health Services
714 P Street
Sacramento, CA 95814
(916) 445-1248

Nonprofit Associations
California Association of Homes for the Aging
7311 Greenhaven Drive, Suite 175
Sacramento, CA 95831
(916) 392-5111

Colorado

Health
Department of Health
4210 E. 11th Avenue
Denver, CO 80220
(303) 331-4600

Aging

Division of Aging and Adult Services
Department of Social Services
State Social Services Building
1575 Sherman Street
Denver, CO 80203
(303) 294-5794

Medicaid

Department of Social Services
1575 Sherman Street
Denver, CO 80203
(303) 294-5800

Nonprofit Associations

Colorado Association of Homes and Services for the Aging
2140 South Holly Street
Denver, CO 80222
(303) 759-8688

Connecticut

Health

Department of Health Services
150 Washington Street
Hartford, CT 06106
(203) 566-2038

Aging

Department on Aging
175 Main Street
Hartford, CT 06106
(203) 566-3238

Medicaid

Department of Income Maintenance
110 Bartholomew Avenue
Hartford, CT 06106
(203) 566-2008

Nonprofit Associations
Connecticut Association of Non-Profit Facilities for the Aged
110 Barnes Road
P.O. Box 90
Wallingford, CT 06492
(203) 269-7443

Delaware

Health
Division of Public Health
Department of Health & Social Services
P.O. Box 637
Dover, DE 19903
(302) 736-4701

Aging
Division of Aging
Department of Health & Social Services
1901 N. DuPont Highway
New Castle, DE 19720
(302) 421-6791

Medicaid
Department of Health & Social Services
Delaware State Hospital
P.O. Box 906
New Castle, DE 19720
(302) 421-6139

District of Columbia

Health
Department of Human Services
Commission of Public Health
1875 Connecticut Avenue, NW
Washington, DC 20009
(202) 673-7700

Aging
Office on Aging
1424 K Street, NW
Washington, DC 20005
(202) 724-5622

Long-Term-Care Administration
Department of Human Services
Commission of Public Health
1660 L Street, NW
Washington, DC 20036
(202) 673-3597

Medicaid
Department of Human Services
801 N. Capitol Street, NE
Washington, DC 20002
(202) 727-0450

Nonprofit Associations
National Capital Area Association of Homes for the Aging
c/o Presbyterian Home
3050 Military Road, NW
Washington, DC 20015
(202) 363-8310

Florida

Health
Health Office
Department of Health and Rehabilitative Services
1323 Winewood Boulevard, Building 1
Tallahassee, FL 32301
(904) 487-2705

Aging
Aging and Adult Services Program Office
Department of Health and Rehabilitative Services
1321 Winewood Boulevard
Tallahassee, FL 32301
(904) 488-8922

Medicaid
Department of Health and Rehabilitative Services
1317 Winewood Boulevard
Tallahassee, FL 32301
(904) 488-7721

Nonprofit Associations
Florida Association of Homes for the Aging
1018 Thomasville Road, #200-Y
Tallahassee, FL 32303
(904) 222-3562

Georgia

Health
Division of Public Health
878 Peachtree Street
Atlanta, GA 30309
(404) 894-7505

Aging
Office of Aging
Georgia Department of Human Resources
878 Peachtree Street
Atlanta, GA 30309
(404) 894-2022

Medicaid
Department of Medical Assistance
2 Martin Luther King Drive, West Tower
Atlanta, GA 30334
(404) 656-4479

Nonprofit Associations
Georgia Association of Homes and Services for the Aging
2719 Burford Highway, Suite 213
Atlanta, GA 30324
(404) 728-0223

Hawaii

Health
Department of Health
1250 Punchbowl Street, P.O. Box 3378
Honolulu, HI 96801
(808) 548-6505

Aging
Executive Office on Aging
335 Merchant Street
Honolulu, HI 96813

(808) 548-2593

Medicaid
Department of Human Services
P.O. Box 339
Honolulu, HI 96809
(808) 548-6260

Idaho

Health
Division of Health
Department of Health and Welfare
450 West State Street
Boise, ID 83720
(208) 334-5945

Aging
Idaho Office on Aging
Statehouse, 700 W. State Street
Boise, ID 83720
(208) 334-3833

Medicaid
Department of Health and Welfare
Statehouse
450 W. State Street
Boise, ID 83720
(208) 334-5500

Illinois

Health
Department of Public Health
535 West Jefferson Street
Springfield, IL 62761
(217) 782-4977

Aging
Department on Aging
421 East Capitol
Springfield, IL 62701
(217) 785-3356

Medicaid
Department of Public Aid
100 S. Grand Avenue E.
Springfield, IL 62762
(217) 782-0963

Nonprofit Associations
Illinois Association of Homes for the Aging
911 North Elm Street, Suite 228
Hinsdale, IL 60521
(312) 325-6170

Indiana

Health
Board of Health
P.O. Box 1964, 1330 W. Michigan Street
Indianapolis, IN 46206
(317) 633-8400

Aging
Division of Aging
251 N. Illinois Street
Indianapolis, IN 46204
(317) 232-1147

Medicaid
State Department of Public Welfare
100 North Senate Avenue
Indianapolis, IN 46204
(317) 232-4705

Nonprofit Associations
Indiana Association of Homes for the Aging
1265 West 86th Street
Indianapolis, IN 46260
(317) 257-1115

Iowa

Health
Department of Public Health
Robert Lucas State Office Building
East 12th & Walnut Streets
Des Moines, IA 50319
(515) 281-5605

Aging
Department of Elder Affairs
914 Grand
Des Moines, IA 50319
(515) 281-5187

Medicaid
Bureau of Medical Services
Department of Human Services
Hoover State Office Building
Des Moines, IA 50319
(515) 281-8794

Nonprofit Associations
Iowa Association of Homes for the Aging
3839 Merle Hay Road, #215
Des Moines, IA 50310
(515) 270-1198

Kansas

Health
Kansas Department of Health & Environment
Forbes Field
Topeka, KS 66620
(913) 296-1522, (ext.) 522

Aging
Department on Aging
620 West 10th Street
Topeka, KS 66612
(913) 296-4986

Medicaid
Department of Social & Rehabilitation Services
State Office Building
Topeka, KS 66612
(913) 296-3271

Nonprofit Associations
Kansas Association of Homes for the Aging
641 S.W. Harrison Street
Topeka, KS 66603
(913) 233-7443

Kentucky

Health
Cabinet for Human Resources
275 East Main Street
Frankfort, KY 40621
(502) 564-3970

Aging
Division for Aging Services
Department for Social Services
Cabinet for Human Resources
275 East Main Street
Frankfort, KY 40621
(502) 564-6930

Medicaid
Department of Medical Assistance
275 East Main Street
Frankfort, KY 40621
(502) 564-4321

Nonprofit Associations
Kentucky Association of Homes for the Aging
Suite #125
1018 South Fourth Street
Louisville, KY 40203
(502) 587-7333

Louisiana

Health
Department of Health and Hospitals
325 Loyola Avenue, P.O. Box 60630
Baton Rouge, LA 70160
(504) 342-6711

Aging
Governor's Office of Elderly Affairs
P.O. Box 80374
Baton Rouge, LA 70898
(504) 925-1700

Medicaid
Department of Health and Hospitals
755 Riverside, P.O. Box 3776
Baton Rouge, LA 70821
(504) 342-6711

Nonprofit Associations
Louisiana Association of Homes and Services for the Aging
2431 South Acadian, Suite 280
Baton Rouge, LA 70808
(504) 928-6894

Maine

Health
Bureau of Health
Department of Human Services
State House Station 11
Augusta, ME 04333
(207) 289-2736

Aging
Bureau of Maine's Elderly
Department of Human Services
State House Station 11
Augusta, ME 04333
(207) 289-2561

Medicaid
Department of Human Services
221 State Street, State House Station 11
Augusta, ME 04333
(207) 289-2736

Maryland

Health
Department of Health and Mental Hygiene
201 West Preston Street
Baltimore, MD 21201
(301) 225-6500

Aging
Maryland Office on Aging
201 West Preston Street
Baltimore, MD 21201
(301) 225-1102

Medicaid
Department of Health and Mental Hygiene
201 West Preston Street
Baltimore, MD 21201
(301) 225-6500

Nonprofit Associations
Maryland Association of Nonprofit Homes for the Aging
6263 Bright Plume
Columbia, MD 21044-3749
(301) 740-4585

Massachusetts

Health
Department of Public Health
150 Tremont Street
Boston, MA 02111
(617) 727-2700

Aging
Department of Elder Affairs
38 Chauncey Street
Boston, MA 02111
(617) 727-7750

Medicaid
Department of Public Welfare
600 Washington Street
Boston, MA 02111
(617) 348-5500

Nonprofit Associations
Association of Massachusetts Homes for the Aging
45 Bromfield Street
Boston, MA 02108
(617) 423-0718

Michigan

Health
Department of Public Health
3500 North Logan Street
Lansing, MI 48909
(517) 335-8024

Aging
Office of Services to the Aging
300 East Michigan
Lansing, MI 48909
(517) 373-7876

Medicaid
Michigan Department of Social Services
P.O. Box 30037
Lansing, MI 48909
(517) 373-2000

Nonprofit Associations
Michigan Nonprofit Homes Association
1615 East Kalamazoo Street
Lansing, MI 48912
(517) 372-7540

Minnesota

Health
Department of Health
717 Delaware Street, SE
P.O. Box 9441
Minneapolis, MN 55440
(612) 623-5460/(612) 623-5463

Aging
Minnesota Board on Aging
Metro Square Building, 7th & Robert Streets
St. Paul, MN 55101
(612) 296-2770

Medicaid
Department of Human Services
444 Lafayette Road
St. Paul, MN 55155
(612) 296-2701

Nonprofit Associations
Minnesota Association of Homes for the Aging
2221 University Ave., SE, #425
Minneapolis, MN 55414
(612) 331-5571

Mississippi

Health
Mississippi State Department of Health
P.O. Box 1700, 2423 North State Street
Jackson, MS 39215
(601) 960-7634

Aging
Council on Aging
421 W. Pascagoula
Jackson, MS 39203
(601) 949-2070

Medicaid
Division of Medicaid
239 N. Lamar Street
Jackson, MS 39201
(601) 359-6050

Missouri

Health
Department of Health
P.O. Box 570
Jefferson City, MO 65102
(314) 751-6001

Aging
Division of Aging
Department of Social Services
P.O. Box 1337
Jefferson City, MO 65102
(314) 751-3082

Medicaid
Department of Social Services
Broadway State Office Building, P.O. Box 1527
Jefferson City, MO 65102
(314) 751-4815

Nonprofit Associations
Missouri Association of Homes for the Aging
6925 Hampton Avenue
St. Louis, MO 63109-3902
(314) 353-9050

Montana

Health
Department of Health and Environmental Sciences
Cogswell Building, Lockey Street
Helena, MT 59620
(406) 444-2544

Aging
Department of Family Services
111 Sanders Street
Helena, MT 59604
(406) 444-3865

Medicaid
Department of Social and Rehabilitation Services
111 Sanders Street, P.O. Box 4210
Helena, MT 59604
(406) 444-5622

Nonprofit Associations
Montana Association of Homes for the Aging
P.O.Box 5774
Helena, MT 59604
(406) 443-1185

Nebraska

Health
Department of Health
301 Centennial Mall South, P.O. Box 95007
Lincoln, NE 68509
(402) 471-2133

Aging
Department on Aging
301 Centennial Mall South, P.O. Box 95044
Lincoln, NE 68509
(402) 471-2306

Medicaid
Department of Social Services
301 Centennial Mall South, P.O. Box 95026
Lincoln, NE 68509
(402) 471-3121

Nonprofit Associations
Nebraska Association of Homes for the Aging
1320 Lincoln Mall, Suite #9
Lincoln, NE 68508
(402) 477-7015

Nevada

Health
Health Division
505 East King Street
Carson City, NV 89710
(702) 885-4740

Aging
Division for Aging Services
505 East King Street
Carson City, NV 89710
(702) 885-4210

Medicaid
Department of Human Resources
505 East King Street
Carson City, NV 89710
(702) 885-4730

New Hampshire

Health
New Hampshire Division of Public Health Services
Health & Welfare Building
6 Hazen Drive
Concord, NH 03301
(603) 271-4501

Aging
Division of Elderly and Adult Services
6 Hazen Drive
Concord, NH 03301
(603) 271-2751

Medicaid
Department of Health and Welfare
6 Hazen Drive
Concord, NH 03301
(603) 271-4334

Nonprofit Associations
Northern New England Association of Homes and Services for
the Aging
c/o Hunt Community
10 Allds Street
Nashua, NH 03060
(603) 882-6511

New Jersey

Health
Department of Health
CN 360
Trenton, NJ 08625
(609) 292-7837

Aging
Department of Community Affairs
Division on Aging
South Broad & Front Streets, CN 807
Trenton, NJ 08625
(609) 292-4833

Medicaid
Department of Human Services
222 South Warren Street, CN 700
Trenton, NJ 08625
(609) 292-3717

Nonprofit Associations
New Jersey Association of Non-Profit Homes for the Aging, Inc.
Box CN 1
Princeton, NJ 08540
(609) 452-1161

New Mexico

Health
Health Services Division
Health and Environment Department
P.O. Box 968
Santa Fe, NM 87503
(505) 984-0030

Aging
State Agency on Aging
Chamisa Hills Building
440 St. Michael's Drive
Santa Fe, NM 87503
(505) 827-7640

Medicaid
Department of Human Services
P.O. Box 2348
Santa Fe, NM 87504
(505) 827-4072

New York

Health
Department of Health
Tower Building, Empire State Plaza
Albany, NY 12237
(518) 474-2011

Aging
New York State Office for the Aging
Empire State Plaza, Agency Building 2
Albany, NY 12223
(518) 474-4425

Medicaid
State Department of Social Services
40 North Pearl Street
Albany, NY 12243
(518) 474-9475

Nonprofit Associations
New York Association of Homes and Services for the Aging
194 Washington Avenue, 4th Floor
Albany, NY 12210
(518) 449-2707

North Carolina

Health
Department of Human Resources
Division of Health Services
P.O. Box 2091
Raleigh, NC 27602
(919) 733-3446

Aging
Department of Human Resources
Division on Aging
Kirby Building, 1985 Umbstead Drive
Raleigh, NC 27604
(919) 733-3983

Medicaid
Department of Human Resources
325 N. Salisbury Street
Raleigh, NC 27611
(919) 733-4534

Nonprofit Associations
North Carolina Association of Nonprofit Homes for the Aging
1717 Park Drive
Raleigh, NC 27605
(919) 821-0803

North Dakota

Health
Department of Health & Consolidated Laboratories
State Capitol
Bismarck, ND 58505
(701) 224-2372

Aging
Aging Services
State Capitol, Judicial Wing
Bismarck, ND 58505
(701) 224-2577

Medicaid
Department of Human Services
State Capitol Building
Bismarck, ND 58505
(701) 224-2310

Nonprofit Associations
North Dakota Nursing Home Association
312-17 1st Bank of ND, Box 669
Grand Forks, ND 58201
(701) 772-4111

Ohio

Health
Ohio Department of Health
246 North High Street
Columbus, OH 43266
(614) 466-2253

Aging
Department of Aging
50 West Broad Street
Columbus, OH 43266
(614) 466-5500

Medicaid
Department of Human Services
30 East Broad Street
Columbus, OH 43215
(614) 466-6282

Nonprofit Associations
Association of Ohio Philanthropic Homes and Housing for the
Aging
36 West Gay Street
Columbus, OH 43215
(614) 221-2882

Oklahoma

Health
Department of Health
1000 N.E. 10th Street, P.O. Box 53551
Oklahoma City, OK 73152
(405) 271-4200

Aging
Department of Human Services
P.O. Box 25352
Oklahoma City, OK 73125
(405) 521-3646

Medicaid
Department of Human Services
P.O. Box 25352
Oklahoma City, OK 73125
(405) 521-3646

Oregon

Health
State Health Division
1400 S.W. 5th Avenue
Portland, OR 97201
(503) 229-5032

Aging
Senior Services Division
313 Public Service Building
Salem, OR 97310
(503) 378-4728

Medicaid
Department of Human Resources
318 Public Service Building
Salem, OR 97310
(503) 378-3034

Nonprofit Associations
Oregon Association of Homes for the Aging
7150 SW Hampton Street, #206
Tigard, OR 97223
(503) 684-3788

Pennsylvania

Health
Department of Health
802 Health & Welfare Building
Harrisburg, PA 17120
(717) 787-6436

Aging
Department of Aging
Barto Building, 231 State Street
Harrisburg, PA 17101
(717) 783-1550

Medicaid
State Department of Public Welfare
Health & Welfare Building
Seventh and Forster Streets
Harrisburg, PA 17120
(717) 787-2600

Nonprofit Associations
Pennsylvania Association of Non-Profit Homes for the Aging
P.O. Box 698
3425 Simpson Ferry Road
Camp Hill, PA 17011
(717) 763-5724

Puerto Rico

Health
Department of Health
Building A, Call Box 70184
San Juan, PR 00936
(809) 766-1616

Medicaid
Department of Health
Building A, Call Box 70184
San Juan, PR 00936
(809) 766-2200

Rhode Island

Health
Department of Health
Cannon Health Building, 75 Davis Street
Providence, RI 02908
(401) 277-2231

Aging
Department of Elderly Affairs
79 Washington Street
Providence, RI 02903
(401) 277-2894

Medicaid
Department of Human Services
600 New London Avenue
Cranston, RI 02920
(401) 464-2121

Nonprofit Associations
Rhode Island Association of Facilities for the Aged
c/o St. Clare Home
309 Spring Street
Newport, RI 02840
(401) 849-3204

South Carolina

Health
Department of Health and Environmental Control
2600 Bull Street
Columbia, SC 29201
(803) 734-4880

Aging
Commission on Aging
915 Main Street
Columbia, SC 29201
(803) 734-3203

Medicaid
State Health and Human Services Finance Commission
P.O. Box 8206
Columbia, SC 29202
(803) 253-6100

Nonprofit Associations
South Carolina Association of Non-Profit Homes for the Aging
c/o Presbyterian Home of South Carolina
Musgrove Street Extension
Clinton, SC 29325
(803) 833-5190

South Dakota

Health
Department of Health
525 E. Capitol, Joe Foss Building
Pierre, SD 57501
(605) 773-3361

Aging
Office of Adult Services and Aging
Department of Social Services
Kneip Building
700 Governors Drive
Pierre, SD 57501
(605) 773-3656

Medicaid
Department of Social Services
Kneip Building
700 Governors Drive
Pierre, SD 57501
(605) 773-3165

Nonprofit Associations
South Dakota Association of Homes for the Aging
P.O. Box 639
Sioux Falls, SD 57101
(605) 338-6621

Tennessee

Health
Department of Health and Environment
344 Cordell Hull Building
Nashville, TN 37219
(615) 741-3111

Aging
Commission on Aging
535 Church Street
Nashville, TN 37219
(615) 741-2056

Medicaid
Department of Health and Environment
344 Cordell Hull Building
Nashville, TN 37219
(615) 741-3111

Nonprofit Associations
Tennessee Association of Homes for the Aging
c/o Joseph B. Knowles Home for the Aged
625 Benton Avenue
Nashville, TN 37204
(615) 259-5601

Texas

Health
Texas Department of Health
1100 West 49th Street
Austin, TX 78756
(512) 458-7111

Aging
Texas Department on Aging
210 Barton Springs Road
Austin, TX 78704
(512) 475-2717

Medicaid
Department of Human Resources
P.O. Box 2960
Austin, TX 78769
(512) 450-3030

Nonprofit Associations
Texas Association of Homes for the Aging
720 Brazos Street, Suite 1104
Austin, TX 78701
(512) 477-6994

Utah

Health
Department of Health
288 N. 1460 West, P.O. Box 16700
Salt Lake City, UT 84116
(801) 538-6111

Aging
Division of Aging
150 W. North Temple
Salt Lake City, UT 84103
(801) 538-3910

Medicaid
Department of Health
288 N. 1460 West, P.O. Box 16580
Salt Lake City, UT 84116
(801) 538-6111

Vermont

Health
Department of Health
P.O. Box 70, 60 Main Street
Burlington, VT 05402
(802) 863-7280

Aging
Office on Aging
Waterbury Complex
Waterbury, VT 05676
(802) 241-2400

Medicaid
Agency of Human Services
103 S. Main Street
Waterbury, VT 05676
(802) 241-2220

Virginia

Health
Department of Health
109 Governor Street
Richmond, VA 23219
(804) 786-3561

Aging
Virginia Department for Aging
700 E. Franklin Street
Richmond, VA 23219
(804) 225-2271

Medicaid
Department of Medical Assistance Services
600 E. Broad Street
Richmond, VA 23219
(804) 786-7933

Nonprofit Associations
Virginia Association of Nonprofit Homes for the Aging
4900 Augusta Avenue, #104
Richmond, VA 23230
(804) 353-8141

Washington

Health
Division of Public Health
Department of Social & Health Services
Mall Stop ET 21
Olympia, WA 98504
(206) 753-5871

Aging
Aging and Adult Services
Department of Social & Health Services
Mall Stop HB 11
Olympia, WA 98504
(206) 586-3768

Medicaid
Division of Medical Assistance
Department of Social & Health Services
Mall Stop HB 41
Olympia, WA 98504
(206) 753-1777

Nonprofit Associations
Washington Association of Homes for the Aging
444 NE Ravenna Boulevard, #208
Seattle, WA 98115
(206) 526-8450

West Virginia

Health
Department of Public Health
1800 Washington Street E
Charleston, WV 25305
(304) 348-2971

Aging
Commission on Aging
State Capitol
Holly Grove
Charleston, WV 25305
(304) 348-3317

Medicaid
West Virginia Department of Human Services
Building 6, State Capitol
Charleston, WV 25305
(304) 348-2400

Wisconsin

Health
Division of Health
P.O. Box 309
Madison, WI 53707
(608) 266-1511

Aging
Bureau on Aging
217 S. Hamilton
Madison, WI 53707
(608) 266-2536

Medicaid
Department of Health and Social Services
1 W. Wilson Street, P.O. Box 7850
Madison, WI 53707
(608) 266-3681

Nonprofit Associations
Wisconsin Association of Homes & Services for the Aging
6400 Gisholt Drive, Suite 203
Madison, WI 53713
(608) 222-5086

Wyoming

Health
Health and Medical Services
Hathaway Building
Cheyenne, WY 82002
(307) 777-6464

Aging
Commission on Aging
Hathaway Building
Cheyenne, WY 82002
(307) 777-7986

Medicaid
Department of Health and Social Services
2300 Capitol Avenue
317 Hathaway Building
Cheyenne, WY 82002
(307) 777-6778

SAMPLE ADMISSIONS AGREEMENTS

CALIFORNIA ADMISSIONS AGREEMENT

TABLE OF CONTENTS

* This section requires completion on each admission.

* This section requires completion on each admission.

THIS ADMISSION AGREEMENT IS A LEGALLY
BINDING CONTRACT. PLEASE READ IT IN ITS ENTIRETY
BEFORE SIGNING IT AND BE SURE YOU UNDERSTAND ITS
TERMS.

PAYMENT STATUS: _____ Private _____ Medi-Cal
_____ Medicare _____ Veterans
Administration

The parties to this contract are:
(a) _____ (hereafter
the "facility");
(b) _____ (hereafter
the "Patient") (if signed by other than the Patient, indicate relationship to
Patient: _____);
(c) _____, the
next of kin, sponsoring agency or other payor or payor representative
personally responsible for payment of any portion of charges incurred by
the Patient (hereafter the "Responsible Party"). RESPONSIBLE
PARTY SIGNATURE OTHER THAN AGENT IS NOT
ALLOWED TO BE REQUIRED OR SOLICITED AS A
CONDITION OF ADMISSION FOR MEDI-CAL BENEFICIARIES;
(d) _____, the
Medi-Cal Beneficiary's agent who manages, uses, or controls funds or assets that legally may be used to pay the Patient's share of cost and other
charges not paid for by the Medi-Cal Program (hereafter the "Agent").
The parties agree, on this _____ day of _____,
199 ____ , that beginning upon the _____ day of _____,
199 ____ , the Facility will admit and provide the services specified,
herein to the Patient until the date of the Patient's discharge and that the
Patient and the Responsible Party, if applicable will pay for services
provided by the Facility pursuant to the terms and conditions contained
herein.

I. NONDISCRIMINATION
The Facility welcomes all persons in need of its services
without regard to age, handicap, race, color, national origin, ancestry,
religion or sex and will make no determinations regarding admissions or
discharges based upon such factors.

II. SERVICES AND SUPPLIES INCLUDED.
A. Basic Services
1. Private Pay Patients. Included in the Basic Daily
Rate set forth in Section VII.A. hereof, the Facility will provide each
private pay Patient with general nursing care as ordered by a physician,
treatment, room, board, clean linens, bedding equipment and shared

facilities and such other services as listed in Schedule A hereto. The supplies and items listed in Schedule A hereto will be furnished for the use of the Patient, in brands to be determined in the discretion of the Facility, at no extra charge to the Patient, his or her family, an Agent and/or the Responsible Party. Upon request of the Patient, additional services and supplies may be provided to the Patient. However, the Patient, Responsible Party and the Agent shall be responsible for paying for such goods or services.

 Personal laundry services are available at the current posted monthly rate. The Facility shall not be responsible for normal deterioration of clothing caused by routine washing. The Facility does not provide dry cleaning or ironing services. If the Patient, or the Responsible Party desire that laundry services be provided to the Patient, the Patient, or the Responsible Party shall initial on the line provided:

——————— .

 If the Patient does not elect to utilize the Facility's laundry services, the Patient and the Responsible Party agree to maintain a plastic container which is equipped with a tight-fitting lid which is marked with the Patient's name and words "Soiled Linen." Patient and Responsible Party agree, for purposes of infection control, to deposit all soiled clothing into said container and to empty said container and to launder the clothes therein at least every other day, and, upon failure to do so, the Facility shall be authorized to take charge of the Patient's laundry needs as if Patient had requested the Facility's laundry service, and to charge the Patient its monthly laundry fee.

 The Patient may elect to be provided by the Facility with optional supplies or services set forth in Schedule C hereto. Patients will receive monthly statements itemizing all charges incurred by them.

 2. <u>Medi-Cal Beneficiaries</u>. The Facility will provide Medi-Cal beneficiaries with all services required to be provided by law to Medi-Cal beneficiaries at no extra charge, including those services described in Title 22, California Administrative Code Sections 51123(a) and 51511(b) or any successor regulations thereto. The Facility will not be responsible for providing those goods or services listed in Title 22, California Administrative Code Sections 51123(b), 51511(c) or 51511(d) or any successor regulations thereto. A copy of Medi-Cal covered services is attached hereto as Schedule B and is incorporated herein by this reference. A copy of optional Medi-Cal supplies and services is attached hereto as Schedule D and is incorporated herein by this reference.

 The Patient and the Agent acknowledge that the goods and services covered by the Medi-Cal program may change from time to time by action of the California or federal governments and that currently covered goods and services accordingly could be considered not to be covered in the future. The Facility will provide the Patient with notice of any such changes.

The Facility will provide standard equipment and furnishings for the Patient's use. If the Patient's attending physician orders special equipment, such equipment will be supplied by the Facility only upon payment of the Facility's direct and indirect costs of providing such equipment if payment for such equipment is not made by the Medi-Cal program.

The Patient may elect to be provided by Facility with goods or services set forth in Schedule D hereto not covered by the Medi-Cal program. Patients will receive monthly statements itemizing all optional charges incurred by them. However, the Patient shall be responsible for paying the direct and incidental costs incurred by the Facility in providing such goods or services.

3. <u>Medicare Beneficiaries</u>. The services and supplies to be provided to the Patient by the Facility are those set forth by federal law as being covered by the Medicare Program. Current services covered under the Medicare Program are set forth in Schedule D attached hereto. Services and supplies not covered may be provided to the Patient upon request. The Patient or the Responsible Party shall be responsible for paying for such goods and services.

B. <u>Private Duty Personnel</u>. The Patient may utilize private duty personnel if use of such personnel is approved in advance by the Facility's administrator. All private duty personnel shall comply with all policies and procedures of the Facility. Failure of private duty personnel to follow such policies and procedures will result in their being denied access to the Facility. Patient, Responsible Party, and/or Agent shall be solely responsible for the cost of private duty personnel.

C. <u>Personal Items</u>. The Patient, Responsible Party or Agent shall provide the Patient with personal comfort items, clothing, and petty cash for the Patient's incidental expenses. All clothing and other personal items shall be clearly marked to indicate that the Patient is the owner thereof.

D. <u>Uncovered Medical Services</u>. If the Patient's physician determines that services are medically necessary which are not provided by the Facility pursuant to this Agreement, payment for such services is the responsibility of the Patient, Responsible Party and/or Agent. If the Patient, Responsible Party or Agent refuses to authorize such services or payment therefor, the Patient, Responsible Party and Agent release the Facility from any and all liability for harm which may result to the Patient due to the lack of such services.

III. <u>CONSENT TO TREATMENT</u>.

A. <u>Nursing Services</u>. The Patient acknowledges that he or she is under the medical treatment and care of an attending physician, and that the Facility renders services to the Patient under the general and specific instructions of said physician. The Patient hereby consents to the Facility providing such routine nursing care as may be directed by said attending physician.

CALIFORNIA ADMISSIONS AGREEMENT *(cont.)*

B. <u>Attending Physician</u>. The Facility will permit the Patient to use the attending physician of the Patient's choice, so long as that professional agrees to abide by the rules and regulations of the Facility and relevant federal and state governments. If the Patient does not select an attending physician, the Patient may request that an attending physician be selected by the Facility. The Patient, Responsible Party or Agent shall be solely responsible for payment of any charges of an attending physician selected by the Facility. The Facility may obtain the services of the attending or a substitute physician when necessary and at least once each 30 days to provide orders for the Patient's care. The Patient agrees that the Facility may require the use of another licensed health care professional if the attending physician is barred from practice in the Facility due to repeated violations of the Facility's rules and regulations, or if any emergency requires an immediate response to the Patient's medical needs with another professional's services.

C. <u>Independent Contractors</u>. The Patient, Responsible Party and Agent recognize and agree that all physicians, including physicians arranged for by the Facility, furnishing services to the Patient are independent contractors and are not employees or agents of the Facility and that the Facility is accordingly not legally responsible for the acts or omissions of such physicians. The Patient, Responsible Party or Agent acknowledge that they are jointly and severally financially liable and responsible for all services rendered by such physicians.

D. <u>Incompetency of Patient</u>. The Patient requests that the Facility contact _____ to assist in making necessary decisions regarding the Patient's care by the Facility when the Patient may be incapable of making such decisions.

E. <u>Right to Refuse Treatment</u>. Patients have the right to refuse treatment to the extent permitted by law and to be informed of the medical consequences of such refusal.

IV. <u>PATIENT'S MEDICAL RECORDS</u>.

A. <u>Confidentiality</u>. Information contained in the Patient's medical records is confidential, and disclosure to unauthorized persons will not be made without written consent, except as required or permitted by law. Authorization for such disclosure is attached as Attachment 1.

B. <u>Consent to Disclosure to Facility</u>. The Patient authorizes any and all skilled nursing facilities, intermediate care facilities, hospitals, or physicians to furnish to the Facility, the Social Security Administration, the California Department of Health Services and all fiscal intermediaries and carriers all requested information from the Patient's medical or financial records.

C. <u>Consent to Disclosure by Facility</u>. The Patient authorizes the Facility to disclose all or any part of the Patient's medical or financial records to any person or entity which is or may be liable under contract to the Facility, to the Patient, or to a family member of employer of the Patient to pay all or a portion of care provided to the

Patient, including, but not limited to, hospital or medical services companies, insurance companies, Worker's Compensation carriers, welfare funds, or the Patient's employer.

   D. Patient Access. Patient has the right to obtain access to his or her health care records in accordance with the Facility's procedures. Forms to be used by Patient in requesting access to such records shall be available from the Facility's administrator.

  V. TRANSFERS OF PATIENTS.

   The Patient and the Responsible Party agree that the Facility from time to time may change the room assignment of the Patient as it may in its discretion determine to be efficient for providing care to the Patient or otherwise appropriate.

   The Facility shall have the right in its discretion to transfer the Patient to a hospital which has a transfer agreement with the Facility if it determines that such transfer is appropriate in order to meet the Patient's needs for health care services.

   The Facility agrees that before transferring the Patient to any other location within or outside of the Facility it will give reasonable advance written notice to the Patient, Responsible Party and/or the Agent, stating the reason for the transfer except when an emergency requires an immediate transfer.

  VI. THE PATIENT'S DUTIES.

   A. Rules and Regulations. The Patient agrees that the Facility may, to maintain economical and orderly operations, adopt reasonable rules and regulations to govern the Patient's behavior. The Patient agrees to obey those rules or regulations and acknowledges that he or she has been given a written copy of such rules or regulations. It is understood that changing circumstances may require changes in these rules and regulations, but any changes will be provided to the Patient in writing before taking effect. Furthermore, there is a Facility Procedure for suggesting changes in the rules and a Facility grievance procedure for resolution of resident complaints about Facility practices. Copies of both procedures shall be available from the Administrator. Patients have the right to contact the State Department of Health Services or the long-term care ombudsman, or both, regarding grievances against the Facility.

   B. Smoking. Because smoking is demonstrably unhealthy, the Patient agrees to refrain from smoking any form of tobacco or other substance except in the facility's designated smoking areas and as expressly permitted by the rules of the Facility, and then only when it is not injurious to the health or welfare of others. The Patient, Responsible Party and Agent agree that the Facility shall not be responsible for any injury which may result to the Patient or the Patient's property as a result of the Patient's smoking. The Patient, Responsible Party and Agent agree to indemnify and hold harmless the Facility against any damages or liability to persons or property which may occur as a result of the Patient's smoking.

C. Diet. The Patient understands that the diet of the Facility's patients is medically prescribed and therefore must be monitored by the Facility. The Patient therefore agrees that he or she will not bring any food or beverages into the Facility without permission from the Facility.

D. Medications. No medications or drugs may be brought upon the Facility's premises unless the medications or drugs are labeled properly. All such medications must be brought to the nurses station. The Facility shall not require patients to purchase drugs, or rent or purchase medical supplies or equipment, from any particular pharmacy or other source. Notwithstanding the foregoing, the Facility may require that controlled substances which are periodically counted by the Facility on at least a daily basis be dispensed by the Patient's pharmacy in containers suitable for that purpose. Nothing in this paragraph shall prevent the Facility from requiring the Patient's pharmacy or other source from complying with the Facility's policies and procedures reasonably necessary for the care of the Patient or required to meet the intent of state or federal regulations.

E. Appliances. Because of fire and other safety concerns, the patient understands that appliances of any kind may not be brought into the Facility without the prior written permission of the Facility. The Patient and the Responsible Party release the Facility from any responsibility for, and agree to indemnify and hold the Facility harmless against, any claims made by the Patient or by other persons with respect to burns, injuries or property damage which may occur as a result of the Patient's use of electrical appliances.

F. Personal Property. The Facility shall make reasonable efforts to safeguard the Patient's property and valuables that are in the possession of the Patient. However, the Patient acknowledges that the Facility may most effectively safeguard the personal property of the Patient only if the Facility has possession of and control over such property. Therefore, the Patient agrees to store all valuable personal property in the Facility's safe or other secured storage area as the Facility may provide. The Facility will not be liable for either damages to or loss of personal property of the Patient except with respect to damage to or as required by law. Effective April 1, 1988 the Facility shall implement a theft and loss program pursuant to Health and Safety Code Section 1289.4. Attachment 6 sets forth the parameters of the theft and loss program.

G. Care of Facility's Property. In order to preserve the value of the Facility's property for future patients' use, the Patient agrees to use due care to avoid damaging the Facility's property or premises. No pictures, posters or other ornaments may be hung on walls, nor may furniture be rearranged in the Patient's room without the prior consent of the administrator of the Facility. The Patient will be responsible for repair or replacement of the Facility's property damaged or destroyed by the Patient. However, the Patient will not be responsible for such damage as is to be expected as ordinary wear and tear.

VII. FINANCIAL ARRANGEMENTS.

A. Private Pay Patients.

1. Daily Rate. The Patients understands that in order to offer quality health care services, the Facility must remain financially sound. The Patient understands that the Facility's basic daily rate is _____ Dollars ($ _____). This daily rate is determined in part by the type of room assigned to the Patient and therefore may be changed if the Patient is transferred to a different room. A charge in the amount of the basic daily rate will be made for the date of admission but not for the day of discharge, except that a late discharge fee in the amount of the agreed basic daily rate will be charged if the Patient fails to vacate his room by 12:00 noon on the date of discharge. The Patient and the Responsible Party agree to pay a sum equal to thirty times the daily rate in advance. Any unused advance payment shall be refunded if the Patient converts to Medi-Cal coverage.

2. Rate Adjustment. It may become necessary, because of inflation or other factors, to increase the daily rate or optional service charges. The Patient will receive no less than thirty (30) days' written advance notice of all rate adjustments as required by law, except as provided by Section 1288(b) of the Health and Safety Code. If at any time the Patient's condition requires a change in the level of care, the Facility will make such a change and adjust the Patient's daily rate accordingly. At each notification of a rate adjustment, the Patient can elect to terminate this Agreement. Any rate increase will be deemed agreed to by both Patient and Responsible Party upon the mailing of said notice unless the Facility is notified in writing to the contrary within ten (10) days after the mailing of the notice of the rate increase. If the Patient and the Responsible Party do not agree to the rate increase, the Patient agrees to leave the Facility no later than the day before the rate increase becomes effective. if the Patient fails to so vacate the Facility, the Patient and the Responsible Party shall be deemed to have consented to the rate increase.

3. Extra Services and Supplies. The Patient and Responsible Party shall be responsible for payment of all charges of the Facility for supplies or services which are not included in the Facility's daily rate.

B. Medi-Cal Patients.

1. Basic Payment. The Patient's basic services as delineated by Section II.A.2 hereof will be provide for payment made under the Medi-Cal program administered by the State of California. Services which are not covered by Medi-Cal must be paid for by the Patient or the Patient's Agent or the Responsible Party (if applicable).

2. Medi-Cal Eligibility. Neither the Patient, Responsible Party nor Agent may be required to pay privately for any period during which the Patient has been approved for payment by

212

Medi-Cal. Pursuant to Welfare and Institutions Code Section 14019.3, upon presentation of a medical card or other proof of eligibility the facility shall submit reimbursement claims to Medi-Cal. And and all payments made by or on behalf of the Patient shall be returned by the Facility upon receipt of Medi-Cal payment provided however any monies legally owing to the Facility and not paid for by the Medi-Cal program shall be retained by the Facility before any monies are returned to the Patient or Agent.

3. Termination of Coverage. The Patient may remain in the Facility only so long as certified eligible for Medi-Cal payments, and as long as any charges owed by the Patient are paid as due. Residents who remain beyond the expiration of their Medi-Cal coverage or who have their coverage retroactively terminated or denied shall be obligated to pay their account as private paying patients with rates and charges for services rendered at the regular rates and terms in effect at the time of the services.

4. Duration of Stay Prohibition. No Medi-Cal certified Facility may require in writing or orally, as a condition of admission, a promise prior to signing this agreement that a Patient will remain in private pay status for a specified period of time.

5. Patient's Share of Cost. The Medi-Cal program determines the monthly income available for all persons receiving Medi-Cal assistance and, with respect to most Medi-Cal beneficiaries, determines a reasonable share of cost, payment of which is the responsibility of the Patient. The Patient's share of cost is subject to change as authorized by law. The Patient agrees to pay his or her share of cost as determined pursuant to the Medi-Cal program. If the Patient fails to make prompt payment of his or her share of cost, the Facility may require direct deposit of such monies with separation of the Patient's personal funds as required by law. The Patient acknowledges that failure to pay the Patient's share of cost constitutes grounds for discharge of the Patient.

C. Medicare Patients.

1. Basic Payment. The Patient's basic services as delineated by Section II.A.3 hereof will be provided for payment made under the Medicare program. Services which are not covered by Medicare must be paid for by the Patient or the Responsible Party.

2. Limited Coverage. The Patient and the Responsible Party understand that Medicare coverage is established by federal guidelines. Under the current Medicare guidelines, the Patient is allowed a maximum of 100 days' stay in the Facility. However, based upon Medicare criteria, Medicare coverage can be terminated at any time prior to the expiration of 100 days.

3. Expiration of Benefits. Evidence of the Patient's ability to pay for care in the Facility upon the expiration of the Patient's Medicare benefits as either a private pay patient or otherwise must be provided by the Patient prior to admission by the Facility in order to

ensure the ability of the Facility to retain the Patient after the expiration of Medicare benefits. If the Patient's or the Responsible Party's intent upon the admission of the Patient is that the Patient be discharged from the Facility upon termination of Medicare coverage, the Patient or Responsible Party shall so notify the Facility at the time of the Patient's admission. The Patient and the Responsible Party agree to pay the Facility's daily rate for thirty days in advance, upon the Patient's changing to private pay status. No payment in advance is required with respect to Patients who convert from Medicare to Medi-Cal coverage.

D. Obligations to Pay. The Patient's account shall be billed monthly to the Patient, Responsible Party or Agent.

E. Due Date. Bills not paid promptly are in default. The Patient, the Responsible Party and the Agent acknowledge that the Facility does not grant credit or allow installment payments. Partial payment is not acceptable under any circumstances. Payment must be made by the fifteenth (15th) of every month, or the Patient's account will be assessed a delinquency charge at the monthly rate of one and one-half percent (1½) (or, if less, the maximum amount permitted by law). The Patient acknowledges that such delinquency charge shall not give the Patient any right to make payments other than within the periods otherwise required hereunder or constitute a forbearance by the Facility of obligations of the Patient. Rather, such delinquency charge represents liquidated damages payable to the Facility agreed by the Patient to be reasonable in light of the impracticability and extreme difficulty of determining the actual damages to the Facility.

F. Failure to Pay. In the event that the Patient, Responsible Party or the Agent fails to make required payments within the period provided, the Facility may require the Patient to vacate the Facility. A reasonable period will be provided to allow the Patient, the Responsible Party or the Agent to make arrangements for the Patient's vacating the Facility. The Patient, Responsible Party and the Agent agree the Patient will vacate the Facility on the date specified by the Facility under this section. The Patient, Responsible Party or Agent will be responsible for all relocation expenses, as well as the daily rate charges due for all days of care received.

G. Insurance Coverage. The Patient, Responsible Party or Agent shall be primarily responsible for making payments pursuant to this paragraph notwithstanding any insurance coverage and shall be responsible for paying all charges not paid by any insurer, including any coinsurance or deductible amounts required by any insurer.

H. Other Payors. The Facility makes no assurance of any kind whatsoever that the Patient's care will be covered by Medicare, Medi-Cal or private insurance companies. The Patient, Responsible Party and Agent hereby release the Facility and its agents and employees from any liability or responsibility in connection with any claim payment by Medicare, Medi-Cal or private insurers.

I. Returned Checks. A Service Fee of $ _____ will be charged for any returned check.

VIII. FACILITY'S MEDI-CAL PARTICIPATION.

The Facility (does/does not) participate(s) in the Medi-Cal program.

IX. TERMINATION OF AGREEMENT.

A. Right To Terminate. No Patient may be transferred or evicted from the Facility solely as a result of the Patient changing his or her manner of purchasing services from private payment or Medicare to Medi-Cal. No Patient can or will be discharged from the Facility except under the following circumstances:

1. Voluntary. A discharge may occur if the Patient elects to leave the Facility, or upon the request of the Responsible Party. Should the Patient leave the Facility before the attending physician discharges the Patient, the Patient agrees to assume all responsibility for all results which may follow.

2. Involuntary. The Facility shall have the right to discharge the Patient if the Patient (1) behaves in a manner disturbing to other patients or does not prevent his or her family or visitors from acting in a manner which is disturbing to other patients, or (2) endangers the health and welfare of patients and staff, or (3) has a diagnosis which does not permit care in the Facility, or (4) has not maintained full current payment of his or her account, or (5) fails to abide by the Facility's reasonable rules of Patient conduct such that his or her or other patients' welfare is endangered, or (6) is a Medi-Cal beneficiary who becomes ineligible for Medi-Cal participation and does not thereafter make payments as a Private Pay Patient, or (7) is a Medi-Cal beneficiary who fails to pay his or her share of the cost, or (8) is no longer in need of nursing care, or (9) provides false information to the Facility as described in Paragraph XVI.D. of this Agreement.

Except in emergencies, the Facility shall give the Patient thirty (30) days' advance written notice of his or her discharge, stating the reason for the discharge. With respect to discharges resulting from nonpayment, the Facility shall give the Patient reasonable advance written notice also stating the reason for the discharge.

B. Refund. If the Patient is discharged before using up the entirety of any prepaid charges, a refund of the unused portion of such charges will be made within fourteen days of the discharge of the Patient. Patient funds which are required by law to be held by the Facility in a demand trust account will be refunded within three banking days of the Patient's date of discharge.

C. Property of Patient Upon Termination. The Facility will attempt to safeguard the Patient's personal belongings, but is not liable for any damage or loss to the Patient's property and will dispose of any belongings left behind by the Patient if not claimed within thirty days of discharge or transfer.

X. <u>BED-HOLDS</u>.

The Patient may request the Facility to hold open the Patient's bed and room while the Patient is absent from the Facility for temporary stays in an acute care hospital. However, except as provided below, the Facility shall have no obligation to hold open the Patient's bed unless it so agrees in writing.

If the Patient is transferred to a general acute care hospital, the Facility shall offer the Patient a bed-hold of seven days which may be exercised by the Patient or by a representative of the Patient. The Patient or the Patient's representative must notify the Facility within twenty-four (24) hours from receipt of notice of bed-hold from the Facility as to whether the Patient wishes to exercise his or her right to a bed-hold. The Facility shall not be required to offer a bed-hold if the Patient requires a level of care greater than that provided by the Facility upon the Patient's return to the Facility. In the event the Facility fails to follow this procedure, the Facility shall offer the next available appropriate bed to the Patient.

Any private pay Patient exercising his or her right to maintain a bed-hold shall pay the Facility's daily rate for the period of that bed-hold. The Patient's insurance may or may not cover the cost of a bed-hold. The Medi-Cal program will reimburse the Facility for up to seven (7) bed-hold days. If Medi-Cal coverage for a bed-hold does not exist, the bed-hold will be considered to be a non-covered service and the Patient shall be obligated to pay the Facility's daily private rate for each day of the bed-hold. The Medicare program does not make payments for bed-holds. Any Medicare Patient exercising his or her right to maintain a bed-hold shall pay the Facility's private daily rate during the period of any bed-hold.

If the Patient's attending physician notifies the Facility in writing that the Patient's treatment at a general acute care hospital will exceed seven days from the date of admission, the Facility shall not be required to maintain a bed-hold for the Patient. If the Patient is transferred from the Facility and does not request a bed-hold or wishes to return to the Facility after the expiration of a requested bed-hold, the Facility shall have no obligation to readmit the Patient.

XI. <u>VISITORS</u>.

Residents shall be permitted to have visitors during established visiting hours. For the safety of the Patient and others, if any of the Patient's guests fail to abide by the Facility's rules for visitors, the Patient and the Responsible Party agree, upon the Facility's request, to arrange for the prompt removal of such visitors from the Facility.

XII. <u>INJURIES TO PATIENT</u>.

The Patient understands that the Facility is liable only for injuries to the Patient caused by the negligent acts or omissions of the Facility or its employees or agents and as required by law.

XIII. TELEPHONE.

A public telephone is provided for use by all patients. If a Patient desires a private phone, he or she may make arrangements directly with the telephone company after first notifying the Facility. The Facility is not responsible for any charges incurred as a result of the Patient's private telephone.

XIV. PATIENT'S RIGHTS UNDER FEDERAL AND STATE LAW.

A. Patient Bill of Rights.

The Facility agrees to abide by the Patient's Bill of Rights. A copy of this bill of rights is attached as Attachment 4 hereto. By signature hereto, Patient acknowledges that he or she has been informed about the Patient's Bill of Rights.

_____

Patient/Responsible Party or Agent

B. Medical Education.

The Patient recognizes that, while he or she has the right to privacy in medical treatment and personal care, the Facility may from time to time become involved in medical education programs through which future health care professionals gain experience. The Facility will always assure that medical treatment is rendered only at the direction of competent licensed professionals and instruct such students as may be involved that all such treatment is confidential and private. The Patient hereby consents to such involvement unless he or she, by later specific writing, denies permission to student health care professionals to become involved in the Patient's treatment.

C. Photographs.

The Patient agrees to permit the Facility to make photographs of the Patient for identification use by staff or for health care purposes. These photographs may be used to help locate the Patient in the event of unauthorized absence from the Facility, but will be otherwise kept confidential. The Patient agrees that the Facility may make photographs of the Patient to document the Patient's physical and medical condition at the time of admission and to thereafter make photographs to document care given to the Patient by the Facility. The Facility shall obtain Patient Authorization on Attachment 3 for use of Patient photographs for other than identification or health care purposes.

XV. RESPONSIBLE PARTY AND/OR AGENT.

A. Responsible Party.

Except with respect to any Medi-Cal beneficiary, it is required that a Responsible Party act as agent and sponsor for the Patient. The Patient and the Responsible Party agree jointly and severally to assume and be liable for all charges of whatever nature incurred by or on behalf of the Patient and to pay such charges as they become due.

The Patient and the Responsible Party understand that if the Patient's stay at the Facility is covered by any insurance, it is nevertheless the joint and several obligation of the Patient and the Responsible Party to pay all charges incurred by or on behalf of the Patient. The Patient and the Responsible Party further understand that any coinsurance or deductible obligation under Medicare or private insurance must be satisfied by the Patient and/or the Responsible Party. The Responsible Party agrees to assume responsibility for the Patient upon the discharge or transfer of the Patient.

NO MEDI-CAL BENEFICIARY SHALL BE REQUIRED TO HAVE AS A CONDITION OF ADMISSION A RESPONSIBLE PARTY SIGN OR CO-SIGN THIS AGREEMENT. If the Patient is a Medi-Cal beneficiary who does not have a Responsible Party, references herein to a Responsible Party shall be disregarded. However, a person may voluntarily assume the obligations of a Responsible Party hereunder with respect to a Medi-Cal beneficiary. If the Patient is not admitted initially as a Medi-Cal beneficiary but converts to Medi-Cal coverage, the obligations of the Responsible Party shall thereafter be null and void unless the Responsible Party agrees to continue to act in such capacity or unless the Responsible Party is in fact the Agent, as defined below, of the Patient, in which case the Responsible Party will continue to have the obligations of the Agent.

B. Medi-Cal Agent.

For purposes of this Agreement, the term "Agent" shall mean any person who manages, uses, or controls funds or assets which may legally be used to pay the Patient's share of costs and/or other charges not paid for by the Medi-Cal program. If the Patient has an agent, such Agent shall be required to sign this Agreement as a condition of the Patient's admission. The Agent's signing of this Agreement signifies his or her agreement to distribute to the Facility when due the Patient's share of cost and any other charges not paid for by the Medi-Cal program which the Patient or the Agent has agreed to pay. The financial obligations of the Agent shall be limited to the amount of the Patient's funds received or held by the Agent, but not distributed to the Facility. Any Agent who willfully violates the above requirements shall be guilty of a misdemeanor and, upon conviction thereof, may be punished by a fine not to exceed two thousand five hundred dollars or by imprisonment in the county jail not to exceed one hundred and eighty days or both.

XVI. ENFORCEMENT.

A. Sole Agreement.

This Agreement, except as specific reference is made to other documents which are attached herein or incorporated herein by reference, is the entirety of the agreement between the Facility and the Patient. Should changes in federal or state law render any part of the Agreement invalid, the remainder of the contract shall stand as a valid agreement.

     B. Acknowledgment.

        By signing below, the Patient and the Responsible Party and/or Agent indicate that they have read the Agreement, clarified any doubts as to its meaning or the meaning of any terms therein, and freely consent to be legally bound by all of its terms and their subsequent implementation by the rules and regulations permitted under this Agreement.

     C. Attorneys' Fees.

        In the event that a legal action should be commenced by any party to this Agreement, including any disputes arising from this Admission Agreement, the prevailing party shall be entitled to recover his or her reasonable costs, including attorneys' fees, incurred in defending or prosecuting such action.

     D. Guarantee of Truthfulness.

        The Patient, Responsible Party and Agent hereby certify and warrant that all information that they have submitted in connection with the Patient's admission, including all information provided in the Patient Information Profile and all information submitted for purposes of applying for or receiving benefits under Title XVIII of the Social Security Act (Medicare) or under Title XIX of said Act (Medicaid), as the case may be, is true and correct.

        The Patient and the Responsible Party understand that the Facility will rely upon the information provided in the Patient Information Profile and other information regarding the Patient's assets and liabilities provided by the Patient, Responsible Party or Agent at the Facility's request in connection with the Patient's admission in making its determination as to whether the Patient shall be admitted to the Facility and that the Facility would not admit the Patient to the Facility but for the accuracy and truthfulness of such information. The Patient understands that he or she may be discharged by the Facility at any time within ninety (90) days of the Patient's date of admission if the Facility discovers that any such information is materially different than represented or omitted by the Patient, Responsible Party or the Agent regardless of whether such misrepresentation or omission could have been discovered earlier by the Facility. In addition, the Facility may initiate discharge of a Patient up to eighteen months from the date of such Patient's date of admission if the Patient has fraudulently misrepresented his or her financial condition so that if the material facts were known by the Facility at the time of the Patient's admission, the Patient would not have been admitted and the Facility could not have discovered the misrepresentation earlier with the exercise of reasonable diligence.

Upon receipt of any notice of discharge for material difference or fraudulent misrepresentation, the Patient may file a complaint with the Office of the State Long-Term Care Ombudsman or State Department of Health Services.

E. Agreement Not Assignable.

The Patient and the Responsible Party acknowledge that the right of the Patient to reside at the Facility is personal and is not assignable.

XVII. NOTICES.

All notices shall be deemed sufficiently served if mailed to the Responsible Party or the Patient at the address set forth below. In addition, the Facility will notify Patient's designee when there is any significant change in the Patient's condition.

The Patient designates the following persons to be notified:

Name: _____   Relationship: _____

Address: _____
           Street   City   State   Zip

Telephone: (_____) _____   (_____) _____
                   Residence   Business

Notification—Medical Information: _____

Non-Medical: _____

OR

Name: _____   Relationship: _____

Address: _____
           Street   City   State   Zip

Telephone: (_____) _____   (_____) _____
                   Residence   Business

Notification—Medical Information: _____

Non-Medical: _____

OR

Name: _____   Relationship: _____

Address: _____
           Street   City   State   Zip

Telephone: (_____) _____   (_____) _____
                   Residence   Business

Notification—Medical Information: _____

Non-Medical: _____

XVIII. MAIL.

The Patient authorizes the Facility to handle the Patient's mail as follows:

_____ All mail directed to the Patient.

_____ The Facility shall forward the Patient's mail to:

_____ Personal mail to the Patient, all business mail to:

_____

Patient or Legal Guardian

Facility Administrator or Designee

_____

Responsible Party (Not required for Medi-Cal)

_____

Agent (For Medi-Cal if applicable)

_____

Street Number

_____

City, State, Zip Code

_____

Telephone

If this Agreement is not signed in the presence of the Facility Administrator or the Facility Administrator's designee, the signatures of the Patient or the legal guardian of the Patient, Agent and the Responsible Party must be notarized.

If the Patient is unable to sign because of legal incompetence or his or her medical condition, the admitting physician shall document the reason in the Patient's medical record.

SCHEDULE A

Supplies and Services Included In the
Private Pay Daily Rate Charge

Room and Board
Routine Nursing Care
Activity Program
Routine Supplies & Equipment (limited to the following):
PLEASE SEE ATTACHED FORM.

SCHEDULE B

Medi-Cal Covered Services

The following services are included in the Medi-Cal rates for intermediate and skilled nursing care:

Room and Board

Routine Nursing Care

Activity Program

Supplies and Equipment (listed below)

<u>Included</u> Supplies and Equipment are:

Autoclaves

Analgesics (non-legend)

Antiseptics

Applicators

Beds

Bed Rails

Bedside Utensils (such as bedpans, basins, irrigating cans, and drinking tubes)

Canes

Charting supplies and other supplies and equipment used in providing intermediate and skilled nursing care

Cradles

Crutches

Footboards

Forceps

Flashlights

First Aid Supplies (such as alcohol, merthiolate, bandages, etc.)

Gauze Dressings

Hair Trims, Periodic

Hypodermic Syringes and Needles

Incontinence Supplies

Infrared Lamps

Irrigating Solutions (Only Sodium Chloride)

Irrigating Standards

Icebags

Laundry, Personal

Laxatives (non-legend)

Lubricants

Mattresses

Nail Files

Oxygen (all equipment necessary for the administration of oxygen other than nasal catheters and than nasal catheters and positive pressure apparatus.)

Patient Lifts

Patient Examining Equipment

Rubbing Compounds

Rubber Goods (such as rectal tubes, catheters, gavage tubing, soft restraints, incontinence pads, urine bags, colostomy or ileostomy pouches and accessories)

Shaves and shampoos performed as part of patient care.

Sterilizers

Scissors

Trapeze Bars

Thermometers

Tongue Depressors

Wheelchairs

Walkers

Weighing Scales

OPTIONAL SUPPLIES AND SERVICES FOR MEDI-CAL BENEFICIARIES

ITEM	CHARGE
ALOE SKIN CREME - 8oz.	6.76
BABY OIL 16oz.	3.25
BABY POWDER 4oz.	2.17
COMB, MAN	.55
COMB, WOMAN	.55
DENTURE CUP (various styles)	.75 to 2.27
DEODORANT, ROLL ON	3.46
FACIAL TISSUE	.75
GUEST MEALS	2.50
INTENSIVE CARE LOTION - 3.5oz.	3.26
MINERAL OIL	3.15
MOUTHWASH 4oz.	2.21
RAZOR, DISPOSABLE	.55
SHAMPOO, BABY 16 oz.	2.97
SHAVE CREAM	2.58
TISSUE WIPES	.55
TOOTHBRUSH	.49

PLEASE NOTE THAT THERE ARE SOME PHARMACY ITEMS THAT ARE NOT PAID BY MEDI-CAL. IF A PATIENT HAS A ZERO SHARE OF COST, THESE PHARMACY ITEMS WILL BE BILLED DIRECTLY TO THE PATIENT OR RESPONSIBLE PARTY.

SCHEDULE C

Optional Supplies and Services for Private Pay Patients

ITEM	CHARGE
Personal Laundry	
Beauty Shop:	
Shampoo	Current charges posted in
Set	the Beauty Shop.
Cut	
Perm	
Color	
Personal Grooming Supplies	*Charge List available from Office Manager.
TV Rental	N/A
Incontinent Supplies	supplied by family
Other	
Medical Supplies and Equipment	*Charge List available from Office Manager.
Physical Therapy*	Charge List available from Office Manager.
Occupational Therapy*	Charge List available from Office Manager.
Speech Therapy*	Charge List available from Office Manager.
Radiology*	Charge List available from Office Manager.
Laboratory*	Charge List available from Office Manager.

*May be billable to Medicare Part B if eligible.

SCHEDULE D

Optional supplies and Service for Medi-Cal Beneficiaries

ITEM	CHARGE
Beauty Shop:	Charges posted in Beauty Shop.
Shampoo	
Set	
Cut	
Permanent Wave	
Coloring	
Personal Grooming Supplies	Charges available from Office Mgr.
Television Rental	N/A

(To be given to the Patient at time of admission and upon conversion to Medi-Cal status.)

SCHEDULE E

Medicare Services

These Medicare charges include the following services:
Room and Board
Routine Nursing Care
Routine Supplies and
  Equipment
Activity Program
Medicare reimbursement <u>includes</u> charges for the following Ancillary Services.

Pharmacy	Physical Therapy
Radiology	Speech Pathology Services
Laboratory	Occupational Therapy
Medical Supplies, Chargeable	

Medicare Reimbursement <u>does not include</u> charges for the following personal needs items or services:

Personal Laundry	Transportation
Personal Grooming Supplies	Equipment Rental
Private Room	Television Rental
Private Duty Nurse	Beauty Shop/Barber Shop Services

Medicare pays 100 percent of the daily room rate plus all ancillary charges for the first 20 days of a benefit period. For each Medicare-covered day thereafter you are required to pay a portion of the charge. That portion is called coinsurance. The coinsurance amount is _____ for 19 _____ .

Medicare will not pay for personal items or services. You will be charged for these and also for the difference between a private and semi-private room if you request a private room. When you are no longer covered for Medicare inpatient services, Medicare will pay 80 percent of the following ancillary services you require, but you will be billed 20 percent coinsurance:

Physical Therapy	Prosthetic Devices
Speech Pathology Services	Radiology
Surgical Dressings	

MEDICAID might pay a portion of Medicare coinsurance for inpatient and outpatient services and supplies. A list of all charges are available for review upon request.

ত

MEDICARE SERVICES COVERED

ROUTINE SERVICES SUCH AS . . . .
- SEMI-PRIVATE ROOM
- ALL MEALS, INCLUDING SPECIAL DIETS
- NURSING CARE AND SUPPLIES
- SOCIAL REHABILITATION (activities)
- SOCIAL SERVICE COORDINATOR
- RESTORATIVE NURSING
- PHARMACY
- MEDICAL SUPPLIES
- LAB, X-RAY, EKG
- OXYGEN

SERVICES WHEN MEDICARE GUIDELINES ARE MET . . . . .
- PHYSICAL THERAPY
- OCCUPATIONAL THERAPY
- SPEECH THERAPY
- RESPIRATORY THERAPY
- CLINITRON THERAPY

Please note that Medicare pays 100% of covered services for first 20 days of benefit period. For the remaining 80 days of benefit period, $65.00 per day coinsurance (1987 rate) is paid by the patient or responsible party.

NON-COVERED SERVICES

PRIVATE ROOM, UNLESS MEDICALLY NECESSARY
PRIVATE DUTY NURSES
PERSONAL CONVENIENCE ITEMS SUCH AS BARBER AND
  BEAUTY, PERSONAL NEED ITEMS

❧

Optional Supplies and Services for Private Pay Patients

ITEM	CHARGE
ABSORPTION DRESSING	8.44 to 39.57
ACE BANDAGE (various sizes)	3.00 to 7.49
ACETEST - 100	20.40
*ACETIC ACID IRRIG-2000cc	17.99
*ACETIC ACID IRRIG-500cc	9.71
ALOE SKIN CREME - 8oz	6.76
APPLICATOR (various sizes)	.08
BABY OIL 16oz.	3.25
BABY POWDER 4oz	2.17
BETADINE SOLUTION (various size bottles)	1.64 to 6.68
BETADINE SWAB STICKS (10)	2.34
BIOCLUSIVE DRESSING (various sizes)	8.40 to 12.96
*CATHETER ALL PURPOSE 14FR or 16FR	1.20
*CATHETER CARE KIT	6.76
*CATHETER PLUG/PROTECTOR	1.99
*CATHETER TRAY, FOLEY	8.60 to 11.61
*COLOSTOMY POUCH (10)	28.22
COMB, MAN	.55
COMB, WOMAN	.55
COMPOSITE PAD	1.02
CONNECTION TUBE (various sizes)	7.22 to 9.03
DECUBITUS PAD	53.04
DENTURE CUP	.75 to 2.27
DEODORANT, ROLL ON	3.46
DOUCHE UNIT, DISPOSABLE	2.02
DRESSING TRAY	13.05
DUO-DERM DRESSING	7.16
EGGCRATE PAD 4″ 34x75	29.68
EGGCRATE PROTCTV SLEEVE	7.80
ENEMA BAG	2.80
ENEMA BUCKET	3.04
ENTERAL NUTR. SUPP. FEEDING (NO NG TUBE)	2.06 to 3.87
EXAM GLOVE	.74 to 1.00
*EXTERNAL CATHETER, K-94	2.18
FACIAL TISSUE	.75
*FOLEY CATH (various sizes and styles)	2.94 to 27.02
GAUZE BANDAGE (various sizes)	.99 to 3.50
GAUZE SPONGE (various sizes)	.54 to .67
GEL FOAM PAD W/COVER	40.88
GUEST MEALS	2.50
HAIRBRUSH, WOMAN	1.50

ITEM	CHARGE
HEEL PROTECTOR	12.22
HEEL/ELBOW/KNEE PROTCTR	15.84
HUMIDIFIER OXYGEN DISP	8.00
HUMIDIFIER PREFILLED DISP	11.01
HYDRO PAD	35.99
INCONTINENT SUPPLIES - DISP (to be supplied by family)	
INTENSIVE CARE LOTION - 3.5oz	3.26
*IRRIGATION SOD. CL. (various size bottles)	9.23 to 11.98
*IRRIGATION SYRINGE	2.45
IRRIGATION TRAY	4.51
*IRRIGATION, WATER (various sizes)	9.36 to 10.99
KERLIX BANDAGE (various sizes)	3.20 to 3.68
LAUNDRY, PERSONAL	20.00
MINERAL OIL	3.15
MINERAL OIL ENEMA, DISP	2.40
MOUTHWASH 4oz.	2.21
NASAL CANULA - OXYGEN	1.60
OP-SITE DRESSING (various sizes)	5.16 to 10.35
OXYGEN	30.00
OXYGEN MASK	3.49
OXYGEN TUBING	2.76
PHOSPHATE ENEMA 4.5oz DISP	1.90
POVIDONE IODINE OINT 16oz	20.88
RAZOR, DISPOSABLE	.56
RESTON PAD - HIGH SUPPORT	9.51
RESTON PAD - MED SUPPORT	6.98
SHAMPOO, BABY 16oz	2.97
SHAVE CREAM	2.58
*STOMA ADHESIVE WAFER (5)	25.34
*STOMACH TUBE (various sizes)	1.82 to 4.02
SUCTION CATH	2.52
SUTURE REMOVAL SET	5.16
SYRINGE & NEEDLE (various sizes and types)	1.25 to 1.89
SYRINGE, DISPOSABLE (various sizes and types)	1.20 to 1.92
TELFA PAD (various sizes)	1.77 to 2.91
TISSUE WIPES	.55
TOOTHBRUSH	.49
TOOTHPASTE, 3.0oz	2.70
URETHRAL CATHETER	2.15
*URINARY DRAINAGE BAG (various sizes)	4.99 to 6.83
VIGILON	3.76
VITAMIN A&D OINT (various sizes)	3.49 to 8.50

ITEM	CHARGE
WATER MATTRESS PURCHASE	74.49
WHEELCHAIR CUSHION	8.22
ZINC OXIDE OINT 16oz.	7.60

*PART B ITEM - 80/20 SPLIT, 80% to Medicare and 20% to private pay patient

☙

JOSEPH L. MORSE GERIATRIC CENTER
ADMISSIONS AGREEMENT

THE JOSEPH L. MORSE GERIATRIC CENTER
4847 Fred Gladstone Drive
West Palm Beach, Florida 33417
(305) 471-5111

RESIDENT'S NAME: _____

DATE OF ADMISSION:_____

Application for the admission of the above named Resident having been made to The Joseph L. Morse Geriatric Center (hereinafter referred to as the "Facility"), the undersigned hereby guarantees to the Facility, payment for services rendered to and on behalf of said Resident.

Charges shall be at the prevailing rates for basic services listed below. Extra charge services are noted and will be billed directly to the undersigned party.

BASIC SERVICES

1. Lodging in a clean, healthful, secure and properly equipped environment.

2. Board, including therapeutic or modified diets as prescribed by a physician.

3. Nursing services, 24 hours per day.

4. Physician services, provided in the Facility.

5. Use of all equipment, medical supplies and modalities, notwithstanding the quantity usually used in the everyday care of Residents, including but not limited to catheters, hypodermic syringes and needles, irrigation outfits, dressings and pads, and so forth.

6. Fresh bed linens as required (and changed by staff) including sufficient quantities of necessary bed linen, or appropriate substitutes changed as often as required for incontinent Residents.

7. Service of holding monies in trust for the safekeeping of Resident's personal funds.

8. Social Services as needed.

9. Assistance and/or supervision, when required, with activities of daily living, including, but not limited to, toileting, bathing, feeding and ambulation assistance.

10. Routine Resident Care Services in the daily performance of their assigned duties, by members of the Facility's staff.

11. Use of customarily stocked equipment, including but not limited to, wheelchairs, walkers and other supportive equipment, including training in their use when necessary.

12. General household medicine cabinet and personal hygiene supplies, including but not limited to non-prescription medications, materials for routine skin care, oral hygiene, care of hair and so forth.

13. Specific medications indicated and prescribed for a specific Resident by an attending physician.

14.   Leisure time activities program seven days per week including, but not limited to, a planned, scheduled program of diverse and meaningful activities together with necessary materials and supplies and assistance with participation therein.

15.   Air conditioning/heat control for each room.

16.   Physical therapy as prescribed by a physician and approved by Medicare, administered by or under the supervision of a licensed and registered physical therapist.

17.   Occupational therapy, as prescribed by a physician and approved by Medicare, administered by or under the supervision of a licensed and currently registered occupational therapist.

18.   Speech therapy, as prescribed by a physician and approved by Medicare, administered by a licensed and currently registered speech pathologist.

19.   Respiratory therapy, as prescribed by a physician and approved by Medicare, administered by a licensed and currently registered respiratory therapist.

20.   Podiatry and Dental services as needed.

21.   Religious services provided in the Facility.

22.   Use of all lounge and outdoor areas.

EXTRA CHARGE SERVICES (See Attached Rate Schedule)

1. Beautician/Barber Shop services.
2. Private In-Room telephones as arranged by the Resident with the local telephone company.

TERMS AND CONDITIONS:

1. Payment in full will be required on the first day of each month. Accounts will be considered in good standing when/if payment is received no later than the 10th day of each month.
2. Billing will be done monthly and will be considered pre-payment for services to be rendered.
3. Refunds will be given on a pro-rated basis in cases when Resident dies or is permanently discharged.
4. Bed holds will be granted upon request at the full daily rate and as per the Facility's Bed Hold Reservation Policy, or the Department of Health and Rehabilitation Service Policy for Medicaid recipients.
5. This contract will be terminated upon a change in Resident's source of payment status.
6. The undersigned party agrees to be solely responsible for payment in full as billed monthly. Unpaid or refusal to pay bills will be grounds for discharge of Resident.
7. The Facility has the absolute right to discharge a Resident provided written notice is given to the undersigned party within twenty four (24) hours of discharge time.
8. The Facility has the right to rate increases provided thirty (30) days written notice is given to the undersigned party.
9. The Facility will not be responsible for provisions of burial, either financially or in any other way.

ॐ

THE JOSEPH L. MORSE GERIATRIC CENTER
ADMISSIONS AGREEMENT *(cont.)*

It is expressly understood that the Facility will accept as payment for services provided the amount of $ _____ per day, to be paid in accordance with the terms and conditions as outlined in the Agreement. The responsible party providing payment will be:

_____

Name   Relationship   Address & Telephone No.

The Facility has the right to bill and accept Medicare Reimbursement for services rendered when applicable.

This Agreement commences on _____, 19_____, and will remain in effect for a minimum of _____ .

_____   _____

Signature of Responsible Party   Facility Administrator

_____   _____

Date   Date

❧

BEAUTY / BARBER SHOP

RATE SCHEDULE

Shampoo and Set	$ 7.00
Haircut (men or women)	6.50
Permanent Waves	25.00/30.00
Single Process Tint	6.00
Weekly Rinses	1.00
Hair Conditioners	1.00/1.50
Manicures	5.00

PRIVATE TELEPHONE

	Rate Schedule
Rent	$13.00 per month
Installation	$36.00
Long Distance Calls	Extra

ADMISSION AGREEMENT

ABC Nursing Home, Inc., and _____hereby agree

Resident or Responsible Party

to the following terms for the nursing and personal care of _____

Resident's Name

NURSING HOME AGREEMENT

1. The management of this facility agrees to exercise such reasonable care toward this person as his or her known condition may require.
2. The facility provides nursing care on a non-discriminatory basis. All residents are admitted and receive services without regard to race, religion, color, sex, age, handicap or national origin.
3. All residents must be admitted per doctor's orders. Prior to admission all residents must have a physical examination according to the period of time determined by the designated level of care and the facility be furnished a copy of the examination.
4. The facility requires that each private pay patient be examined at least annually by his or her physician and a report be provided for the patient records.
5. The facility will not admit or retain addicts, alcoholics, maternity cases, persons having or suspected of having communicable diseases or mental or physical conditions endangering others or themselves.
6. The facility reserves the right to limit admissions or recommend Discharge Transfer if administration deems the resident requires social, emotional, medical and nursing care that cannot be adequately provided by the staff of this facility. Except in an emergency, the facility will provide 5 days written notice to appropriate parties, (i.e., resident/responsible party, attending physician) when such care can no longer be provided. The notice will specify the following: reason for proposed transfer, effective date of transfer and other facilities that may be available.
7. Charges for all services or supplies will be itemized on monthly billing. Payment due by the 10th of every month. Any willful destruction of facility property will be charged by separate billing.

AGREEMENT OF RESIDENT AND RESPONSIBLE PARTY

1. To arrange for the services of an attending physician and a designated alternate to be contacted in the event the attending physician is unavailable. The arrangements will include a commitment to see the resident either by visitation in this home or through office visits.
2. To provide written inventory of personal belongings and valuables, in duplicate, upon forms furnished by the nursing home, properly signed by the resident or responsible party at admission. Liability for the security of personal items retained by the resident or in the

resident's room will not be assumed by the facility. It is recommended that personal insurance be carried on items retained by residents in the facility, specifically jewelry.

3. To provide spending money as needed by the resident. Resident or responsible party is responsible for the safekeeping of resident monies.

4. To provide wash and wear clothing, properly marked, in sufficient quantities to keep resident neatly dressed. Clothes must be marked upon admission.

5. To be responsible for hospital and ambulance charges, if hospitalization of resident becomes necessary.

6. To assist with transportation of the resident whenever possible.

7. To be financially responsible for physician's fee, medications, special equipment, oxygen and other treatments or aids ordered by the resident's physician which are not covered by Medicare/Medicaid and/or other special contracts or agreements.

8. To acccept that only one member of the family may have jurisdiction over the admission, care, or discharge of this resident.

9. To refrain from bringing in items not allowed for residents.

10. To assume all financial and legal responsibliity for private duty nurses employed by the resident and or responsible party. All special duty nurses or sitters will be expected to follow the rules and regulations of this home and will be subject to dismissal for violations.

MEDICATIONS/SUPPLIES

1. All medications must be prescribed by a licensed physician and administered by licensed nurses or other persons who have been approved in accordance with state regulations. Arrangements for the purchase of medications will be made when the resident is admitted. The cost will be assumed by the resident's family or agent. Medicaid recipients will not be charged for non-legend drugs; or supplies and equipment which are considered a part of the daily vendor payments. All medications will be under security precaution as required by law or facility policy.

2. Medications allowed in resident rooms are limited to emergency medications as determined by physician orders.

3. All medications must be ordered by the facility and should come direct from the pharmacy to the nursing home. The pharmacy should provide 24-hour service to the resident.

4. Medications, including controlled drugs, will be released to the resident/responsible party at discharge only by order of the attending physician.

SPECIAL ARRANGEMENTS

1. PODIATRIST

   This is your authority to have the above designated resident visited by the podiatrist who currently services this facility, with written permission of the physician.

2. BLANKET RELEASE

   The undersigned resident or responsible party hereby releases the facility, its agents and employees, from all liability in connection with the resident's participation in any activities within the facility, or while away from the facility on special field trips, medical services or other activities, or in the transportation to and from the facility. Permits the facility to photograph the resident for identification purposes.

3. DENTAL AGREEMENT

   This is your authority to have dental or oral hygiene care given to the above designated resident and for the dentist to bill the responsible party direct for any charges.

4. LAUNDRY AGREEMENT

   This is your authority to have personal laundry done by the facility for the above designated resident. Resident will not be charged for personal laundry which can be washed and fluff dried with regular wash and dry process. Dry cleaning must be provided from an outside resource at the expense of the resident and/or responsible party. All clothes must be marked at the time of admission.

5. PHARMACY AGREEMENT

   Each resident has complete freedom of choice in the selection of the pharmacy to provide the resident's medication. The pharmacy should provide 24-hour service and direct delivery. This is your authority to order all medication from _____ Pharmacy and to allow generic substitutions for named brand items in accordance with physician orders.

6. DISCHARGES

   A "Room Hold Reservation" charge will be made if the resident, or responsible party elects to reserve a room during the resident's absence from the home. The rate per day will not exceed the prevailing daily rate.

7. PASSES

   Residents are allowed to leave the premises for passes with permission of the physician and responsible party. The resident, or responsible party, should discuss all passes with nursing service prior to leaving and must sign out at the nursing desk when leaving and sign in when returning. Legend medications may accompany the resident upon order of the attending physician and must be returned to the nurse in charge when returning to the facility. Overnight

passes for Medicaid recipients must be discussed with the
Administrator who will give you the current policy according to the
level of care and/or agency regulations.

8. MEDICAL TRANSPORTATION

The facility will provide normal transportation service to medical services outside the facility when ordered by the physician, and when
transportation is not obtainable from family, friends, sponsors, civic
groups, or charitable organizations. Normal transportation will be the
nearest Title XIX Medical Care provider, as defined in the ICF/SNF
Standards of Participation. This is your authority to bill the resident
or bill me directly for any expenses incurred beyond normal tranport-
ing plus 25¢ a mile with a minimum charge of $15.00.

9. FUNERAL ARRANGEMENTS

In the event of need, I desire that _____
Funeral Home handle the arrangements for the named resident.

10. CONTRIBUTIONS

Medicaid recipient—patient's right to this facility and its nursing
services is not contigent upon contributions.

11. PERSONAL FUNDS

The resident is under no obligation to deposit funds with the facility.
The resident may manage his/her own personal funds or may
authorize one of the following designees to hold and safeguard these
personal funds.

Representative
    Payee   _____   Other Person _____

    ABC Nursing Home, Inc. _____

FINANCIAL AGREEMENT

The resident and responsible party agree to the rate of $ _____ per day for a _____ room accommodation to be paid one month in advance. $_____ will be paid at the time of admission for the first month's charges. It is understood that this rate may be later adjusted by the facility upon appropriate advance written notice to the resident/responsible party. The charges will be incurred for the day of admission but not for the day of discharge, unless the resident remains in the facility after the established check-out time of 11:00 A.M.

Failure of responsible party to pay for services deemed necessary and proper by the facility, or prescribed by the physician, will release the facility from any and all liability which may result from lack of such services, will be sufficient grounds for the facility to require immediate removal of the resident. Responsible party agrees to transfer resident without delay upon written notice to do so.

REFUNDS

Residents desiring to move shall receive a refund of any unearned portion of the rental of which they are entitled upon request, provided all terms of this agreement have been met. All reasonable efforts will be made to refund by the twentieth (20th) of the month following discharge, provided all monies due or accruing the home have been paid by parties or agents responsible for payment.

* *

_____   _____
Signature of Responsible Party   Signature of Resident

Date:_____   Date:_____

_____   _____
Signature of Nursing Home Rep.   Witness (If Needed)

Date:_____

* *

ACKNOWLEDGMENT OF RESIDENT'S RIGHTS

As a staff member of this facility, I acknowledge that I have reviewed the Resident's Rights document, and that I have further encouraged this resident to ask questions which I have answered to the best of my ability. According to my knowledge I believe that the resident (or where appropriate, the responsible party) understands the intent of each statement contained herein.

_____ Date: _____
Staff Member's Signature

I/We sign this acknowledgment with the understanding that the Resident's Rights benefit the resident's interest and individuality, and further, that they have been explained to me orally and that I have received a copy for my future reference. I have no further questions with regard to the rights of residents in this facility.

_____ Date: _____
Resident's Signature

_____ Date: _____
Responsible Party Signature

FEDERAL REGULATIONS ON RESIDENTS' RIGHTS

(1) GENERAL RIGHTS.—

(A) Specified rights.—A nursing facility must protect and promote the rights of each resident, including each of the following rights:

(i) **Free choice.**—The right to choose a personal attending physician, to be fully informed in advance about care and treatment, to be fully informed in advance of any changes in care or treatment that may affect the resident's well-being, and (except with respect to a resident adjudged incompetent) to participate in planning care and treatment or changes in care and treatment.

(ii) **Free from restraints.**—The right to be free from physical or mental abuse, corporal punishment, involuntary seclusion, and any physical or chemical restraints imposed for purposes of discipline or convenience and not required to treat the resident's medical symptoms. Restraints may only be imposed—

(I) to ensure the physical safety of the resident or other residents, and

(II) only upon the written order of a physician that specifies the duration and circumstances under which the restraints are to be used (except in emergency circumstances specified by the Secretary) until such an order could reasonably be obtained.

(iii) **Privacy.**—The right to privacy with regard to accommodations, medical treatment, written and telephone communications, visits, and meetings of family and of resident groups.

(iv) **Confidentiality.**—The right to confidentiality of personal and clinical records.

(v) **Accommodation of needs.**—The right—

(I) to reside and receive services with reasonable accommodations of individual needs and preferences, except where the health or safety of the individual or other residents would be endangered, and

(II) to receive notice before the room or roommate of the resident in the facility is changed.

(vi) **Grievances.**—The right to voice grievances with respect to treatment or care that is (or fails to be) furnished, without discrimination or reprisal for voicing the grievances and the right to prompt efforts by the facility to resolve grievances the resident may have, including those with respect to the behavior of other residents.

(vii) **Participation in resident and family groups.**—The right of the resident to organize and participate in resident groups in the facility and the right of the resident's family to meet in the facility with the families of other residents in the facility.

(viii) **Participation in other activities.**—The right of the resident to participate in social, religious, and community activities that do not interfere with the rights of other residents in the facility.

(ix) **Examination of survey results.**—The right to examine, upon reasonable request, the results of the most recent survey of the facility conducted by the Secretary or a State with respect to the facility and any plan of correction in effect with respect to the facility.

(x) **Other rights.**—Any other right established by the Secretary. Clause (iii) shall not be construed as requiring the provision of a private room.

(B) **Notice of rights.**—A nursing facility must—

(i) inform each resident, orally and in writing at the time of admission to the facility, of the resident's legal rights during the stay at the facility;

(ii) make available to each resident, upon reasonable request, a written statement of such rights which statement is updated upon changes in such rights;

(iii) inform each resident who is entitled to medical assistance under this subchapter—

(I) at the time of admission to the facility or, if later, at the time the resident becomes eligible for such assistance, of the items and services (including those specified under section 1396a(a)(28)(B) of this title) that are included in nursing facility services under the State plan and for which the resident may not be charged (except as permitted in section 1396o of this title), and of those other items and services that the facility offers and for which the resident may be charged and the amount of the charges for such items and services, and

(II) of changes in the items and services described in subclause (I) and of changes in the charges imposed for items and services described in that subclause; and

(iv) inform each other resident, in writing before or at the time of admission and periodically during the resident's stay, of services available in the facility and of related charges for such services, including any charges for services not covered under subchapter XVIII of this chapter or by the facility's basic per diem charge.

The written description of legal rights under this subparagraph shall include a description of the protection of personal funds under paragraph (6) and a statement that a resident may file a complaint with a State survey and certification agency respecting resident abuse and neglect and misappropriation of resident property in the facility.

(C) **Right of incompetent residents.**—In the case of a resident adjudged incompetent under the laws of a State, the rights of the resident under this title shall devolve upon, and, to the extent judged necessary by a court of competent jurisdiction, be exercised by, the person appointed under State law to act on the resident's behalf.

(D) **Use of psychopharmacologic drugs.**—Psychopharmacologic drugs may be administered only on the orders of a physician and only as part of a plan (included in the written plan of care described in paragraph (2)) designed to eliminate or modify the symptoms for which the drugs are prescribed and only if, at least annually an independent, external consultant reviews the appropriateness of the drug plan of each resident receiving such drugs.

(2) TRANSFER AND DISCHARGE RIGHTS.—

(A) In general.—A nursing facility must permit each resident to remain in the facility and must not transfer or discharge the resident from the facility unless—

(i) the transfer or discharge is necessary to meet the resident's welfare and the resident's welfare cannot be met in the facility;

(ii) the transfer or discharge is appropriate because the resident's health has improved sufficiently so the resident no longer needs the services provided by the facility;

(iii) the safety of individuals in the facility is endangered;

(iv) the health of individuals in the facility would otherwise be endangered;

(v) the resident has failed, after reasonable and appropriate notice, to pay (or to have paid under this subchapter or subchapter XVIII of this chapter on the resident's behalf) for a stay at the facility;

(vi) the facility ceases to operate. In each of the cases described in clauses (i) through (iv), the basis for the transfer or discharge must be documented in the resident's clinical record. In the cases described in clauses (i) and (ii), the documentation must be made by the resident's physician, and in the case described in clause (iv) the documentation must be made by a physician. For purposes of clause (v), in the case of a resident who becomes eligible for assistance under this subchapter after admission to the facility, only charges which may be imposed under this subchapter shall be considered to be allowable.

(B) Pre-transfer and pre-discharge notice.—

(i) **In general.**—Before effecting a transfer or discharge of a resident, a nursing facility must—

(I) notify the resident (and, if known, an immediate family member of the resident or legal representative) of the transfer or discharge and the reasons therefor,

(II) record the reasons in the resident's clinical record (including any documentation required under subparagraph (A)), and

(III) include in the notice the items described in clause (iii).

(ii) **Timing of notice.**—The notice under clause (i)(I) must be made at least 30 days in advance of the resident's transfer or discharge except—

(I) in a case described in clause (iii) or (iv) of subparagraph (A);

(II) in a case described in clause (ii) of subparagraph (A), where the resident's health improves sufficiently to allow a more immediate transfer or discharge;

(III) in a case described in clause (i) of subparagraph (A), where a more immediate transfer or discharge is necessitated by the resident's urgent medical needs; or

(IV) in a case where a resident has not resided in the facility for 30 days.

In the case of such exceptions, notice must be given as many days before the date of transfer or discharge as is practicable.

(iii) **Items included in notice.**—Each notice under clause (i) must include—

(I) for transfers or discharges effected on or after October 1, 1989, notice of the resident's right to appeal the transfer or discharge under the State process established under subsection (e)(3) of this section;

(II) the name, mailing address, and telephone number of the State long-term care ombudsman established under section 3027(a)(12) of this title;

(III) in the case of residents with developmental disabilities, the mailing address and telephone number of the agency responsible for the protection and advocacy system for developmentally disabled individuals established under part C of the Developmental Disabilities Assistance and Bill of Rights Act [42 U.S.C.A. § 6041 et seq.]; and

(IV) in the case of mentally ill residents (as defined in subsection (e)(7)(G)(i) of this section), the mailing address and telephone number of the agency responsible for the protection and advocacy system for mentally ill individuals established under the Protection and Advocacy for Mentally Ill Individuals Act [42 U.S.C.A. § 10801 et seq.].

(C) Orientation.—A nursing facility must provide sufficient preparation and orientation to residents to ensure safe and orderly transfer or discharge from the facility.

(D) Notice on bed-hold policy and readmission.—

(i) Notice before transfer.—Before a resident of a nursing facility is transferred to hospitalization or therapeutic leave, a nursing facility must provide written information to the resident and an immediate family member or legal representative concerning—

(I) the provisions of the State plan under this subchapter regarding the period (if any) during which the resident will be permitted under the State plan to return and resume residence in the facility, and

(II) the policies of the facility regarding such a period, which policies must be consistent with clause (iii).

(ii) Notice upon transfer.—At the time of transfer of a resident to a hospital or for therapeutic leave, a nursing facility must provide written notice to the resident and an immediate family member or legal representative of the duration of any period described in clause (i).

(iii) Permitting resident to return.—A nursing facility must establish and follow a written policy under which a resident—

(I) who is eligible for medical assistance for nursing facility services under a State plan,

(II) who is transferred from the facility for hospitalization or therapeutic leave, and

(III) whose hospitalization or therapeutic leave exceeds a period paid for under the State plan for the holding of a bed in the facility for the resident,

will be permitted to be readmitted to the facility immediately upon the first availability of a bed in a semiprivate room in the facility if, at the time of readmission, the resident requires the services provided by the facility.

(3) ACCESS AND VISITATION RIGHTS.—A NURSING FACILITY MUST—

(A) permit immediate access to any resident by any representative of the Secretary, by any representative of the State, by an ombudsman or agency described in subclause (II), (III), or (IV) of paragraph (2)(B)(iii), or by the resident's individual physician;

(B) permit immediate access to a resident, subject to the resident's right to deny or withdraw consent at any time, by immediate family or other relatives of the resident;

(C) permit immediate access to a resident, subject to reasonable restrictions and the resident's right to deny or withdraw consent at any time, by others who are visiting with the consent of the resident;

(D) permit reasonable access to a resident by any entity or individual that provides health, social, legal, or other services to the resident, subject to the resident's right to deny or withdraw consent at any time; and

(E) permit representatives of the State ombudsman (described in paragraph (2)(B)(iii)(II)), with the permission of the resident (or the

resident's legal representative) and consistent with State law, to examine a resident's clinical records.

(4) EQUAL ACCESS TO QUALITY CARE.—

(A) In general.—A nursing facility must establish and maintain
identical policies and practices regarding transfer, discharge, and the
provision of services required under the State plan for all individuals
regardless of source of payment.

(B) Construction.—

(i) **Nothing prohibiting any charges for non-Medicaid
patients.**—Subparagraph (A) shall not be construed as prohibiting a nursing facility from charging any amount for services furnished, consistent with the notice in paragraph (1)(B) describing
such charges.

(ii) **No additional services required.**—Subparagraph (A) shall
not be construed as requiring a State to offer additional services on
behalf of a resident than are otherwise provided under the State
plan.

(5) ADMISSIONS POLICY.—

(A) Admission.—With respect to admissions practices, a nursing
facility must—

(i) (I) not require individuals applying to reside or residing in
the facility to waive their rights to benefits under this subchapter
or subchapter XVIII of this chapter, (II) not require oral or written assurance that such individuals are not eligible for, or will not
apply for, benefits under this subchapter or subchapter XVIII of
this chapter, and (III) prominently display in the facility written
information, and provide to such individuals oral and written
information, about how to apply for and use such benefits and
how to receive refunds for previous payments covered by such
benefits;

(ii) not require a third party guarantee of payment to the facility as a condition of admission (or expedited admission) to, or continued stay in, the facility; and

(iii) in the case of an individual who is entitled to medical assistance for nursing facility services, not charge, solicit, accept, or receive, in addition to any amount otherwise required to be paid under the State plan under this subchapter, any gift, money, donation, or other consideration as a precondition of admitting (or expediting the admission of) the individual to the facility or as a requirement for the individual's continued stay in the facility.

(B) Construction.—

(i) **No preemption of stricter standards.**—Subparagraph (A) shall not be construed as preventing States or political subdivisions therein from prohibiting, under State or local law, the discrimination against individuals who are entitled to medical assistance under the State plan with respect to admissions practices of nursing facilities.

(ii) **Contracts with legal representatives.**—Subparagraph (A)(ii) shall not be construed as preventing a facility from requiring an individual, who has legal access to a resident's income or resources available to pay for care in the facility, to sign a contract (without incurring personal financial liability) to provide payment from the resident's income or resources for such care.

(iii) **Charges for additional services requested.**— Subparagraph (A)(iii) shall not be construed as preventing a facility from charging a resident, eligible for medical assistance under the State plan, for items or services the resident has requested and received and that are not specified in the State plan as included in the term "nursing facility services."

(iv) **Bona fide contributions.**—Subparagraph (A)(iii) shall not be construed as prohibiting a nursing facility from soliciting, accepting, or receiving a charitable, religious, or philanthropic contribution from an organization or from a person unrelated to the resident (or potential resident), but only to the extent that such contribution is not a condition of admission, expediting admission, or continued stay in the facility.

(6) PROTECTION OF RESIDENT FUNDS.—

(A) **In general.**—The nursing facility—

(i) may not require residents to deposit their personal funds with the facility, and

(ii) upon the written authorization of the resident, must hold, safeguard, and account for such personal funds under a system established and maintained by the facility in accordance with this paragraph.

(B) **Management of personal funds.**—Upon written authorization of a resident under subparagraph (A)(ii), the facility must manage and account for the personal funds of the resident deposited with the facility as follows:

(i) Deposit.—The facility must deposit any amount of personal funds in excess of $50 with respect to a resident in an interest bearing account (or accounts) that is separate from any of the facility's operating accounts and credits all interest earned on such separate account to such account. With respect to any other personal funds, the facility must maintain such funds in a non-interest bearing account or petty cash fund.

(ii) Accounting and records.—The facility must assure a full and complete separate accounting of each such resident's personal funds, maintain a written record of all financial transactions involving the personal funds of a resident deposited with the facility, and afford the resident (or a legal representative of the resident) reasonable access to such record.

(iii) Notice of certain balances.—The facility must notify each resident receiving medical assistance under the State plan under subchapter XIX of this chapter when the amount in the resident's account reaches $200 less than the dollar amount determined under section 1382(a)(3)(B) of this title and the fact that if the amount in the account (in addition to the value of the resident's other nonexempt resources) reaches the amount determined under such section the resident may lose eligibility for such medical assistance or for benefits under subchapter XVI of this chapter.

(iv) Conveyance upon death.—Upon the death of a resident with such an account, the facility must convey promptly the resident's personal funds (and a final accounting of such funds) to the individual administering the resident's estate.

(C) Assurance of financial security.—The facility must purchase a surety bond, or otherwise provide assurance satisfactory to the Secretary, to assure the security of all personal funds of residents deposited with the facility.

(D) Limitation on charges to personal funds.—The facility may not impose a charge against the personal funds of a resident for any item or service for which payment is made under this subchapter or subchapter XVIII of this chapter.

(7) POSTING OF SURVEY RESULTS.—

A nursing facility must post in a place readily accessible to residents, and family members and legal representatives of residents, the results of the most recent survey of the facility conducted under subsection (g) of this section.

BIBLIOGRAPHY

Ambramovice, B. *Long Term Care Administration*. New York: Haworth Press, 1988.

American Association of Retired Persons. *The Right Place and the Right Time*. Washington, DC, 1985.

American Bar Association. *Personal and Estate Planning for the Elderly*. Chicago: American Bar Association, 1989.

American College of Physicians, Health and Public Policy Committee. "Comprehensive Functional Assessment for Elderly Patients." *Annals of Internal Medicine* 109:70–72 (1988).

————. "Financing Long-Term Care." *Annals of Internal Medicine* 108:279–88 (1988).

Andolsek, K.M., et al. "Caregivers and Elderly Relatives." *Archives of Internal Medicine*." 148:2177–80 (1988).

Arling, G.; Nordquist, R.H.; and Capitman, J.A. "Nursing Home Cost and Ownership Type: Evidence of Interaction Effects." *HSR: Health Services Research* 22(2)255–69 (1987).

Avorn, J.; Dreyer, P.; Connelly, K.; and Soumerai, S.B. "Use of Psychoactive Medication and the Quality of Care in Rest Homes." *New England Journal of Medicine* 320(4):227–32 (1989).

Branch, L.G., et al. "Impoverishing the Elderly: A Case Study of the Financial Risk of Spend-Down Among Massachusetts Elderly People." *The Gerontologist* 28(5): 648–52 (1988).

Brody, E.M. "Women in the Middle and Family Help to Older People." *The Gerontologist* 25(1):19–29 (1981).

Champion, H.R., et al. "Major Trauma in Geriatric Patients." *American Journal of Public Health* 79(9):1278–82 (1989).

Cohen, M.A.; Tell, E.J.; Batten, H.L.; and Larson, M.J. "Attitudes Toward Joining Continuing Care Communities." *The Gerontologist* 28(5):637–43 (1988).

Consumer Reports. "Who Can Afford a Nursing Home?" May 1988, 300–311.

Consumer Reports. "Communities for the Elderly." February 1990, 123–131.

Dimant, J. "Beyond the Regulations: Some Thoughts on the Role of the

Medical Director in the Long-Term Care Facility." *Nursing Homes*, January–February 1986, 25–27.

Gallo, J.J.; Reichel, W.; and Andersen, J. *Handbook of Geriatric Assessment*. Rockville, MD: Aspen Publications, 1988.

Goode, J. "Dad's Last Home." *Texas Monthly*, January 1989:106–8.

Goodenough, G.K.; and Goodenough, L.F. "The Recertification Visit: Maximizing the Benefit for the Resident." *Nursing Homes*, March–April 1988, 19–21.

Gutkin, C.E.; and Morris, J. "Changes in Life Status: Improvement, Decline and Nursing Care Effects." Paper presented at the annual meeting of the American Public Health Association, Boston, November 1988.

Haley, S.W. "The Quality Care Pyramid." *Nursing Homes*, July–August 1988, 16–17.

Horn, L.; and Griesel, E. *Nursing Homes: A Citizens' Action Guide*. Boston: Beacon Press, 1977.

Horner, J.M. *That Time of Year: A Chronicle of Life in a Nursing Home*. Amherst, MA: University of Massachusetts Press, 1982.

Institute of Medicine. *Improving the Quality of Care in Nursing Homes*. Washington, DC: National Academy Press, 1986.

Jacobs, B. "Using Home Equity to Finance Long-Term Care." *Journal of Health Politics, Policy and Law*, 12(1):77–95 (1987).

JAMA. "The Teaching Nursing Home: A Golden Annex to the Ivory Tower." *Journal of the American Medical Association* 257(22):3119–20 (1987).

Kalser, L. "Caring For Our Parents," *South Florida Magazine* 42:7 (1989).

Kane, R.A.; and Kane, R.L. *Assessing the Elderly*. Lexington, MA: Lexington Books, 1981.

Kane, R.L.; et al. "Effects of a Geriatric Nurse Practitioner on Process and Outcome of Nursing Home Care." *American Journal of Public Health* 79(9):1271–77 (1989).

Kapp, M.C.; Eichorn, A.M.; and Spector, W.D. "Quality of Care in Nursing Homes: Indicators from New York and Texas." Paper presented at the annual meeting of the American Public Health Association, Boston, November 1988.

Laventhol and Horwath. *Nursing Home Industry 1988*. Philadelphia: Laventhol and Horwath, 1988.

Levey, S.; and Loomba P., eds. *Long-Term Care Administration: A Managerial Perspective* Parts I and II. New York: Spectrum Press, 1977.

Longo, D.R.; Burmeister, R.; and Warren, M. "Do Not Resuscitate: Policy and Practice in the Long-Term Care Setting." *Journal of Long-Term Care Administration*. Spring 1988, 5–11.

Manheim, L.M., and Hughes, S.L. "Use of Nursing Homes by a High Risk Long-Term Care Population." *HSR: Health Services Research* 21(2), 161–76 (1986).

McVey, L.J.; Becker, P.M.; Saltz, C.C.; Feussner, J.R.; and Cohen, H.J. "Effects of Geriatric Consultation Team on Functional Status of Elderly Hospitalized Patients." *Annals of Internal Medicine* 110:(1)79–84 (1989).

Meiners, M.R.; Thorburn, P.; Roddy, P.C.; and Jones, B.J. *Nursing Home Admissions: The Results of an Incentive Reimbursement Experiment*. U.S. Department of Health and Human Services. DHHS Pub. No. (PHS) 86–3397, October 1985.

Meiners, M.R.; and Gollub, J.O. "Long-Term Care Insurance: The Edge of an Emerging Market." *Healthcare Financial Marketing*. March 1984.

Mendelson, M.A. *Tender Loving Greed*. New York: Vintage Books, 1975.

Miller, D.B.; and Barry, J.T. *Nursing Home Organization and Operation*. Boston: CBI Publishing, 1979.

Mohide, E.A.; et al. "A Randomized Trial of Quality Assurance in Nursing Homes." *Medical Care* 26(6)554–65 (1988).

Mongeau, S., ed. *Directory of Nursing Homes*, 3d ed. Phoenix, AZ: Oryx Press, 1988.

Morris, J.N.; Sherwood, S.; May, M.I.; and Bernstein, E. "FRED: An Innovative Approach to Nursing Home Level-of-Care Assignments." *HSR: Health Services Research* 22:(1)117–38 (1987).

Mosher-Ashley, P. "Effects of Family Care on the Placement of the Elderly in Nursing Homes." *Nursing Homes*, July–August 1988, 35–37.

Moss, F.E., and Halamandaris, V.J. *Too Old, Too Sick, Too Bad*. Rockville, MD: Aspen Publications, 1977.

Muller, C. "Homesharing and Congregate Housing." *Research on Aging* 9(2):163–81 (1987).

Munley, A. *The Hospice Alternative*. New York: Basic Books, 1983.

National Center for Health Statistics, G. Strahan. *Nursing Home Characteristics: Preliminary Data from the 1985 National Nursing Home Survey*. Advance Data from Vital and Health Statistics, No. 131. DHHS Pub. No. 87–1250 (1987). Hyattsville, MD: Public Health Service.

National Center for Health Statistics, E. Hing. *Use of Nursing Homes by the Elderly: Preliminary Data from the 1985 National Nursing Home Survey*. Advance Data from Vital and Health Statistics, No. 135. DHHS Pub. No. 87–1250 (1987). Hyattsville, MD: Public Health Service.

National Center for Health Statistics, E.S. Sekscenski. *Discharges from Nursing Homes*. Advance Data from Vital and Health Statistics, No. 142. DHHS Pub. No. 87–1250 (1987). Hyattsville, MD: Public Health Service.

National Center for Health Statistics, A. Sirrocco. *Nursing and Related Care Homes as Reported from the 1986 Inventory of Long-Term Care Places*. Advance Data from Vital and Health Statistics, No. 147. DHHS Pub. No. 88–1250 (1988). Hyattsville, MD: Public Health Service.

National Center for Health Statistics, M.G. Kovar. *Aging in the Eighties, People Living Alone—Two Years Later*. Advance Data from Vital and Health Statistics, No. 149. DHHS Pub. No. 88–1250 (1988). Hyattsville, MD: Public Health Service.

National Center for Health Statistics, G. Strahan. *Characteristics of Registered Nurses in Nursing Homes*. Advance Data from Vital and Health Statistics, No. 152. DHHS Pub. No. 88–1250 (1988). Hyattsville, MD: Public Health Service.

New York State Health Care Committee. *Nursing Home Without Walls Program: A Decade of Quality Care at Home for NY's Aged & Disabled.* Albany, NY, 1988.

Paradis, L.F., ed. *Hospice Handbook: A Guide for Managers and Planners.* Rockville, MD: Aspen Publications, 1985.

Pillemer, K.; and Moore, D.W. "Abuse of Patients in Nursing Homes: Findings from a Survey of Staff." *The Gerontologist* 29(3):314–20 (1989).

Raper, A.T.; and Kalicki A.C., eds. *National Continuing Care Directory: Retirement Communities with Nursing Care,* 2d ed. Glenview, IL: Scott, Foresman & Co., An American Association of Retired Persons Book 1988.

Ray, W.A.; Federspiel, C.F.; Baugh, D.K.; and Dodds, S. "Interstate Variation in Elderly Medicaid Nursing Home Populations." *Medical Care* 25:738–52 (1987).

Regan, J.J. *Your Legal Rights in Later Life.* Glenview, IL: Scott, Foresman & Co., 1989.

Richards, M.; Hooyman, N.; Hansen, M.; Brandts, W.; Smith-DiJulio, K.; and Dahm, L. *Choosing a Nursing Home: A Guidebook for Families.* Seattle: University of Washington Press, 1984.

Roddy, P.C.; Liu, C.K.; and Meiners, M.R. *Resource Requirements of Nursing Home Patients Based on Time and Motion Studies.* U.S. Department of Health and Human Services. DHHS Pub. No. (PHS) 87–3408 (1987). Public Health Service.

Saunders, C.; Summers D.H.; and Teller N., eds. *Hospice: The Living Idea.* Philadelphia: W.B. Saunders, 1981.

Schneider, E., et al., eds. *The Teaching Nursing Home.* New York: Raven Press, 1985.

Schwab, T., ed. *Caring for an Aging World.* New York: McGraw-Hill, 1989.

Shaughnessy, P.W. "Long-Term Care Research and Public Policy." *HSR: Health Services Research* 20(4):489–99 (1985).

Shore, H. "A Resident-Directed Adult Study Program in a Home for the Aged." *Geriatrics* 14:52–55 (1959).

Shore, H. "Programs Which Make a Home a Good Place to Live." *Nursing Home Administrator,* March–April 1962.

Shore, H. "A Kinder, Gentler Old Age." The Goldstein/Fleishman Geriatric Lectureship, presented at the annual meeting of the Jewish Center for the Aged, St. Louis, MO, March 1989.

Shore, H.; Rosenstein, J.; and Wilson, R. "How Administrators of Nonprofit Facilities Size up Their Boards." *Nursing Homes* 31:2–3 (1982).

Smith, D.B. *Long-Term Care in Transition.* Washington, DC: AUPHA Press, 1981.

Solomon, D.H., moderator. "New Issues in Geriatric Care." *Annals of Internal Medicine* 108:718–32 (1988).

Spector, W.D.; and Drugovich, M.L. "Reforming Nursing Home Quality Regulation: Impact on Cited Deficiencies and Nursing Home Outcomes." *Medical Care* 27(8):789–801 (1989).

Tamarkin, C. "A Home Not Her Own." *People,* October 3, 1988, 101–11.

Tedards, W.P. "Quality of Care: The Continuing Development of the PaCS Survey." *Nursing Homes* March–April, 1987, 8–12.

Tellis-Nayak, V. *Nursing Homes Exemplars of Quality.* Springfield, IL: Charles C. Thomas Publishers, 1988.

Thomas, W. *Nursing Homes and Public Policy.* Ithaca, NY: Cornell University Press, 1969.

Townsend, C. *Old Age: The Last Segregation.* New York: Grossman Publishers, 1971.

U.S. Department of Health and Human Services. Proceedings of the Surgeon General's Workshop on Health Promotion and Aging, March 1988.

U.S. General Accounting Office. *Posthospital Care: Discharge Planners Report Increasing Difficulty in Placing Medicare Patients* (GAO/PEMD–87–5BR), 1987. Washington, DC: General Accounting Office.

U.S. General Accounting Office. *Medicaid: Interstate Variations in Benefits and Expenditures* (GAO/HRD–87–67BR), 1987. Washington, DC: General Accounting Office.

U.S. General Accounting Office. *Medicare and Medicaid: Stronger Enforcement of Nursing Home Requirements Needed* (GAO/HRD–87–113), 1987. Washington, DC: General Accounting Office.

U.S. General Accounting Office. *Medicaid: Recoveries from Nursing Home Residents' Estates Could Offset Program Costs* (GAO/HRD–89–56), 1989. Washington, DC: General Accounting Office.

U.S. General Accounting Office. *Medicaid: Some Recipients Neglect to Report Savings Bond Holdings* (GAO/HRD–89–43), 1989. Washington, DC: General Accounting Office.

U.S. General Accounting Office. *Board and Care: Insufficient Assurances That Residents' Needs Are Identified and Met* (GAO/HRD–89–50), 1989. Washington, DC: General Accounting Office.

Vladeck, B. *Unloving Care.* New York: Basic Books, 1980.

Vogel, R.J.; and Palmer H.C., eds. *Long-Term Care Perspectives from Research and Demonstrations.* U.S. Department of Health and Human Services, Health Care Financing Administration, Washington, DC, 1982.

Weissert, W.G. "Hard Choices: Targeting Long-Term Care to the 'At Risk' Aged." *Journal of Health Politics, Policy and Law* 11(3), 464–81 (1986).

Zimmerman, J.M. *Hospice: Complete Care for the Terminally Ill.* Baltimore: Urban and Schwarzenburg, 1986.

INDEX

ABOUT THE AUTHOR

SETH B. GOLDSMITH is Professor of Health Policy and Management at the School of Public Health of the University of Massachusetts at Amherst. He has held academic appointments at Tulane University and Columbia University, where he also served as director of the graduate program in Health-Services Administration. Dr. Goldsmith has served as a member of the New York State Board of Examiners for Nursing-Home Administrators. He is active in the nursing-home field as vice-president of the executive board of a major geriatric center, the Jewish Nursing Home of Western Massachusetts. He was awarded a Robert Wood Johnson Foundation–funded fellowship in long-term-care management. Professor Goldsmith is editor of a professional journal, *Journal of Ambulatory Care Management*, and author and editor of seven textbooks and numerous professional articles. He has also served as a hospital administrator, consultant, and lawyer. He has his M.S. in Hospital Administation from Columbia University, his doctorate from Johns Hopkins University, and his law degree from Western New England College. He practices law with the firm of Bowditch & Dewey in Worcester, Massachusetts.